CATS:
HOMOEOPATHIC REMEDIES

Other works by George Macleod

THE TREATMENT OF HORSES BY HOMOEOPATHY
THE TREATMENT OF CATTLE BY HOMOEOPATHY
A VETERINARY MATERIA MEDICA
DOGS: HOMOEOPATHIC REMEDIES
GOATS: HOMOEOPATHIC REMEDIES
PIGS: THE HOMOEOPATHIC APPROACH TO THE
TREATMENT AND PREVENTION OF DISEASES

CATS:
Homoeopathic Remedies

G. Macleod
MRCVS, DVSM, Vet. FF Hom

RIDER
LONDON • SYDNEY • AUCKLAND • JOHANNESBURG

1 3 5 7 9 10 8 6 4 2

First published in Great Britain
by The C. W. Daniel Company Limited.
Revised editions 1991, 1993, reprinted 1995, 1997, 2001.
This edition published in 2005 by Rider,
an imprint of Ebury Publishing, Random House,
20 Vauxhall Bridge Road, London SW1V 2SA
www.randomhouse.co.uk

Random House Australia (Pty) Limited
20 Alfred Street, Milsons Point, Sydney,
New South Wales 2061, Australia

Random House New Zealand Limited
18 Poland Road, Glenfield,
Auckland 10, New Zealand

Random House South Africa (Pty) Limited
Isle of Houghton, Corner Boundary Road & Carse O'Gowrie,
Houghton 2198, South Africa

The Random House Group Limited Reg. No. 954009

Index compiled by Francesca Garwood-Gowers

Papers used by Rider are natural, recyclable products
made from wood grown in sustainable forests.

Printed and bound by Mackays of Chatham, Chatham, Kent

A CIP catalogue record for this book is available from the British Library

ISBN 1844131947

This book gives non-specific, general advice and should not be relied on as a substitute for proper veterinary or medical consultation. The author and publisher cannot accept responsibility for illness arising out of the failure to seek medical advice from a veterinarian.

Contents

Introduction

This book has been written in the hope that it will satisfy the needs of the many cat lovers who are interested in an alternative approach to the treatment of illnesses to which this endearing species is subject. It is by no means exhaustive and only the common remedies are listed in the text. For a detailed description of remedies the reader is referred to a more comprehensive manual of homoeopathic remedies.

Many of the non-specific conditions mentioned in the text are in many ways similar to those affecting the dog, but it has been found in practice that the response of the cat to any given remedy is different in many respects to that seen in the dog (or other species).

The general format of the text is on the same lines as that which obtains in the author's book on dogs and the short materia medica of the commoner remedies is again the same.

WHAT IS HOMOEOPATHY?

For readers who have little or no knowledge of homoeopathic medicine a brief description of its essentials is necessary to the proper understanding of the role of the remedies in treatment.

Homoeopathy is a branch of medicine which states that any substance which can cause symptoms of illness in man or animal can also be used in the treatment of any condition showing similar symptoms. The principle of likeness between disease condition and remedy is emphasised. If we imagine the illness and the provings of the remedy representing two clinical pictures we should endeavour as far as possible when treating to match one picture against the other. The closer the approximation of the two pictures (the likeness) the more likely we are to achieve satisfactory results in treatment. This is much easier to achieve in human than in veterinary medicine as subjective (mental) symptoms known only to the patient are difficult if not impossible to elicit in animals. Mental symptoms are extremely important in the treatment by homoeopathy in the human patient.

1

Observation of an animal's behaviour and how it reacts to any given situation, to other animals or people, to noise etc. will in some measure compensate for the lack of communication by speech. In certain circumstances it may be possible to imagine how the animal is feeling e.g. the one which may feel grief at the loss of a companion; the one subjected to forced separation from the owner as in quarantine kennels, or those suffering post-operative psychological trauma.

Fortunately the homoeopathic materia medica contains remedies which are helpful in all these instances.

NATURE OF HOMOEOPATHIC REMEDIES

Homoeopathic remedies are obtained from all natural sources, e.g. plant and animal kingdoms and also minerals and their compounds with other chemicals. Homoeopathy is frequently referred to (quite erroneously) as herbal medicine. Nothing could be further from the truth as study of the previous remarks will show. While herbal medicine employs many plants successfully it is unable to exploit the intrinsic merits of plants in the way that homoeopathic medicine is able to do.

PREPARATION OF REMEDIES

Preparation of homoeopathic remedies is a scientific procedure which is best left to a qualified pharmacist trained in the particular techniques. Homoeopathy is too important for remedies to be prepared in any way but the best obtainable. Briefly the system is based on a series of dilutions and succussions (of which more later) which is capable of rendering even a poisonous substance safe to use.

To prepare a potentised remedy a measured drop of a solution called mother tincture (Ø) derived from plant or biological material is added to 99 drops of a water/alcohol mixture and the resultant dilution subjected to a mechanical shock which is called succussion. This process which is essential to the preparation imparts energy to the medium which is rendered stable. One drop to 99 parts water/alcohol

2

mixture is represented by 1c on the centesimal scale. Preparations are also made on the decimal scale and marketed as 1x (on the continent as 1d). Repeated dilutions and succussions yield higher potencies releasing more energy in the process. It will be appreciated therefore that homoeopathy is a system of medicine which concerns itself with energy and not with material doses of a drug.

After a dilution of 3c has been reached which represents 1/100/000 all poisonous or harmful effects of any substance are lost and only the curative properties remain.

SELECTION OF POTENCIES

Once the simillimum or 'most likely' remedy has been selected the question of which potency to use arises. As a general rule in the author's experience the higher potencies which are more energised than the lower should be employed in acute infections or conditions while the lower should be reserved for chronic conditions with or without pathological changes being present. It will be found occasionally that there are exceptions to this point of view and indeed many practitioners especially on the continent rely mostly on lower potencies for general use.

The potencies mentioned under each remedy in the text covering the various diseases are a guide only. Higher potencies than those mentioned will necessitate professional advice.

ADMINISTRATION OF REMEDIES

Remedies are marketed as medicated tablets and powders and also as tinctures and water dilutions. Cats are generally less co-operative than dogs when the need arises for medication and there is no ideal way which will suit every cat.

Owners must determine which system is the best for the particular animal being treated. Some cats readily accept tablets, others powders and others again in liquid form by syringe. Extremely difficult animals can have the remedy incorporated in food or milk and while this is not ideal it has been shown in practice that remedies are equally effective if given in this way.

It is important to avoid subjecting the patient to undue stress and if the patient is unco-operative, the remedy should be given in food.

CARE OF REMEDIES

The delicate nature of the remedies which is inherent in the preparation renders them subject to contamination by strong-smelling substances, e.g. camphor, disinfectants etc. and also by strong sunlight. It is essential therefore that they be kept away from such influences and stored in a cool dry place away from strong light. The use of amber glass bottles is helpful in this connection for storage of tablets.

NOSODES AND ORAL VACCINES

It will be noticed in the text under treatment of various specific conditions that reference is made to the term nosode, and it is necessary to explain fully to what this term refers.

A nosode (from the Greek NOSOS meaning disease) is a disease product obtained from any part of the system in a case of illness and thereafter potentised e.g. cat flu nosode prepared from respiratory secretions of affected cats. In specific, i.e. bacterial, viral and protozoal disease the causative organism may or may not be present in the material and the efficacy of the nosode in no way depends on the organism being present. The response of the tissues to invasion by bacteria or viruses results in the formation of substances which are in effect the basis of the nosode.

An oral vaccine is prepared from the actual organism which causes a disease and may derive from filtrates containing only the exotoxins of the bacteria or from emulsions containing both bacteria and their toxins. These filtrates and emulsions are then potentised and become oral vaccines.

INTRODUCTION

There are two different ways of employing nosodes and oral vaccines.

1. *Therapeutically and* 2. *Prophylactically*

When we employ nosodes therapeutically we may use them for the condition from which the nosode was derived e.g. cat flu nosode in the treatment of a viral rhinotracheitis. This may be termed isopathic, i.e. treatment with a substance taken from an animal suffering from the same disease: or we may employ the nosode in any condition, the symptoms of which resemble the symptom-complex of the particular nosode e.g. the use of the nosode *Psorinum* in the treatment of the particular form of skin disease which appears in the provings of that nosode. This method may be termed homoeopathic i.e. treatment with a substance taken from an animal suffering from a similar disease. In this connection it must be remembered that many nosodes have been proved in their own right, i.e. each has its own particular drug picture. Many veterinary nosodes have been developed but no provings exist for them and they are used almost entirely in the treatment or prevention of the associated diseases.

Autonosodes. This particular type of nosode is prepared from material provided by the patient alone, e.g. pus from a chronic sinus or fistula and after potentisation used for the treatment of the same patient. Many examples of this could be quoted but I think it is sufficient to explain the theory. Autonosodes are usually employed in refractory cases where well indicated remedies have failed to produce the desired response and frequently they produce striking results.

Oral Vaccines. As with nosodes, oral vaccines may be used both therapeutically and prophylactically. If the condition is caused wholly by bacterial or viral invasion the use of the oral vaccine is frequently attended by spectacular success but this is less likely when there is an underlying chronic condition complicating an acute infection. Here we may need the help of constitutional and other remedies.

Bowel Nosodes. The bowel nosodes are usually included under the heading of oral vaccines as the potentised vaccines are prepared from cultures of the organisms themselves. As a preliminary introduction to the study of the bowel nosodes let us consider the role of the E. coli

5

organism. In the normal healthy animal the function of the E. coli bacteria is beneficial rendering complex materials resulting from the digestive process into simpler substances. If however, the patient is subjected to any change, e.g. stress, which affects the intestinal mucosa, the balance between normal health and illness will be upset and the E. coli organisms may then be said to have become pathogenic. This change in the patient need not be a detrimental one, as the administration of potentised homoeopathic remedies can bring it about. The illness therefore may originate, in the patient which causes the bacteria to change their behaviour.

In laboratory tests it has been noticed that from a patient who had previously yielded only E. coli there suddenly appeared a large percentage of non-lactose fermenting bacilli of a type associated with the pathogenic group of typhoid and paratyphoid disease. Since the non-lactose fermenting bacilli had appeared after a latent period of 10 – 14 days following the administration of the remedy it would seem that the homoepathic potentised remedy had changed the bowel flora. The pathogenic germ in this case was the result of vital stimulation set up in the patient by the potentised remedy; the germ was not the *cause* of any change. Each germ or bacillus is associated with its own peculiar symptom-picture and certain conclusions may be made from clinical and laboratory observation. These may be summarised as follows:

a) The specific organism is related to the disease.
b) The specific organism is related to the homoeopathic remedy.
c) The homoeopathic remedy is related to the disease.

The bowel nosodes which concern us in veterinary practice are as follows: 1. Morgan-Bach; 2. Proteus-Bach; 3. Gaertner-Bach; 4. Dys Co-Bach; 5. Sycotic Co-Paterson.

Morgan-Bach. Clinical observations have revealed the symptom-picture of the bacillus Morgan to cover in general digestive and respiratory systems with an action also on fibrous tissues and skin. It is used mainly in eczema of young cats combined with an appropriate remedy, compatible ones being Sulphur, Graphites, Petroleum and Psorinium.

Proteus-Bach. The central and peripheral nervous systems figure prominently in the provings of this nosode, e.g. convulsions and seizures together with spasm of the peripheral circulation: cramping of the muscles is a common feature: angio-neurotic oedema frequently occurs and there is marked sensitivity to ultra-violet light. Associated remedies are Cuprum Metallicum, and Natrium Muriaticum.

Gaertner-Bach. Marked emaciation or malnutrition is associated with this nosode. Chronic gastro-enteritis occurs and there is a tendency for the animal to become infested with worms. There is an inability to digest fat. Associated remedies are Mercurius, Phosphorus and Silicea.

Dys Co-Bach. This nosode is chiefly concerned with the digestive and cardiac systems.

Pyloric spasm occurs with retention of digested stomach contents leading to vomiting. There is functional disturbance of the heart's action, sometimes seen in nervous cats, usually associated with tension.

Associated remedies are Arsenicum Album, Argentum Nitricum and Kalmia Latifolia.

Sycotic Co-Paterson. The keynote of this nosode is sub-acute or chronic inflammation of mucous membranes especially those of the intestinal tract where a chronic catarrhal enteritis occurs. Chronic bronchitis and nasal catarrh are met with.

Associated remedies are Mercurius Corrosivus, Nitricum Acidum and Hydrastis.

MAIN INDICATIONS FOR THE USE OF THE BOWEL NOSODES

When a case is presented showing one or two leading symptoms which suggest a particular remedy we should employ that remedy, if necessary in varying potencies, before abandoning it and resorting to another if unsatisfactory results ensue. In chronic disease there may be conflicting symptoms which suggest several competing remedies and it is here that the bowel nosodes may be used with advantage. A study of the associated remedies will usually lead us to the particular nosode to be employed. The question of potency and repetition of dosage assumes special importance when considering the use of bowel nosodes. The mental and emotional symptoms which are frequently present in illness in the human being are not available to a veterinary surgeon and he therefore concerns himself with objective signs and pathological change. The low to medium potencies, e.g. 6c. – 30c. are more suitable for this purpose than the higher ones and can be safely administered daily for a few days. Bowel nosodes are deep-acting remedies and should not be repeated until a few months have elapsed since the first prescription.

I acknowledge the pamphlet written by the late Dr. John Paterson.

Materia Medica

Abies Canadensis. Hemlock Spruce. N.O. Coniferae.
The Ø is made from the fresh bark and young buds.
  This plant has an affinity for mucous membranes generally and that of the stomach in particular, producing a catarrhal gastritis. Impairment of liver function occurs leading to flatulence and deficient bile-flow. Appetite is increased and hunger may be ravenous. It is chiefly used as a digestive remedy.

Abrotanum. Southernwood. N.O. Compositae.
Tincture of fresh leaves.
  This plant produces wasting of muscles of lower limbs and is used for animals showing this weakness. A prominent guiding symptom in the young animal is umbilical oozing of fluid. It is one of the remedies used to control worm infestation in young animals and also has a reputation in certain forms of acute arthritis where overall symptoms agree.

Absinthum. Wormwood.
Infusions of active principle.
  The effect on the system of this substance is to produce a picture of confusion and convulsions preceded by trembling of muscles. There is a marked action on the central nervous system causing the patient to fall backwards. The pupils of the eye may show unequal dilation. It is one of the main remedies used in practice to control epileptiform seizures and fits of varying kinds.

Acidum Salicylicum. Salicylic Acid.
Trituration of powder.
  This acid has an action on joints producing swellings and in some cases caries of bone. Gastric symptoms e.g. bleeding are also prominent in its provings. Homoeopathically indicated in the treatment of rheumatic and osteo-arthritic conditions and idiopathic gastric bleeding.

9

Aconitum Napellus. Monkshood. N.O. Ranunculaceae.
In the preparation of the Ø the entire plant is used as all parts contain aconitine the active principle.

This plant has an affinity for serous membranes and muscular tissues leading to functional disturbances. There is sudden involvement and tension in all parts. This remedy should be used in the early stages of all feverish conditions where there is sudden appearance of symptoms which may also show an aggravation when any extreme of temperature takes place. Predisposing factors which may produce a drug picture calling for Aconitum include shock, operation and exposure to cold dry winds, or dry heat. It could be of use in puerperal conditions showing sudden involvement with peritoneal complications.

Actaea Racemosa. Black Snake Root. Also referred to as Cimicifuga Racemosa. N.O. Ranunculaceae.
Trituration of its resin.

This plant resin has a wide range of action on various body systems, chief among which are the female genital and the articular leading to disturbances of the uterus in particular and small joint arthritis. Muscular pains are evident, affection of cervical vertebrae are evidenced by stiffening of neck muscles.

Adonis Vernalis. N.O. Ranunculaceae.
Infusion of fresh plant.

The main action of the remedy which concerns us in veterinary practice is its cardial action which becomes weak leading to dropsy and scanty output of urine. It is one of the main remedies used in valvular disease and difficult respiration dependent on pulmonary congestion.

Aesculus Hippocastanum. Horse Chestnut. N.O. Sapindaceae.
The Ø is prepared from the fruit with capsule.

The main affinity of this plant is with the lower bowel producing a state of venous congestion. There is a general slowing down of the digestive and circulatory systems, the liver and portal action becoming sluggish. This is associated with a tendency to dry stools. It is a useful remedy in hepatic conditions with venous congestion affecting the general circulation and it also has a place in the treatment of congestive chest conditions.

10

Agaricus Muscarius. Fly Agaric. N.O. Fungi.
The Ø is prepared from the fresh fungus.

Muscarin is the best known toxic compound of several which are found in this fungus. Symptoms of poisoning are generally delayed from anything up to twelve hours after ingestion. The main sphere of action is on the central nervous system producing a state of vertigo and delirium followed by sleepiness. There are four recognised stages of cerebral excitement. Viz: 1. Slight stimulation. 2. Intoxication with mental excitement accompanied by twitching. 3. Delirium. 4. Depression with soporific tendency. These actions determine its use in certain conditions affecting the central nervous system, e.g. cerebro-cortical necrosis and meningitis, which may accompany severe attacks of hypomagnesaemia. Tympanitic conditions with flatus may respond favourably while it also has a place as a rheumatic remedy and in the treatment of some forms of muscular cramp.

Agnus Castus. Chaste Tree. N.O. Verbenaceae.
Tincture of ripe berries.

One of the principal spheres of action relating to this plant is the sexual system where it produces a lowering or depression of functions with accompanying debility. In the male there may be induration and swelling of testicles and in the female sterility has been reported.

Aletris Farinosa. Star Grass. N.O. Haemodoraceae.
The Ø is prepared from the root.

This plant has an affinity with the female genital tract, especially the uterus and is used mainly as an anti-abortion remedy and in the treatment of uterine discharges and also in silent heat in animals which may show an accompanying loss of appetite.

Allium Cepa. Onion. N.O. Liliaceae.
The Ø is prepared from the whole plant.

A picture of coryza with acrid nasal discharge and symptoms of laryngeal discomfort is associated with this plant. It could be indicated in the early stages of most catarrhal conditions producing the typical coryza.

Alumen. Potash Alum.
Trituration of the pure crystals.

Indicated in affections of limbs and in conditions affecting mucous membranes of various body systems, producing dryness: affections of the central nervous system are also common, resulting in varying degrees of paralysis.

Ammonium Carbonicum. Ammonium Carbonate.
This salt is used as a solution in distilled water from which the potencies are prepared.

It is primarily used in respiratory affections especially when there is an accompanying swelling of associated lymph glands.

Ammonium Causticum. Hydrate of Ammonia.
Potencies are again prepared from a solution in distilled water.

This salt has a similar but more pronounced action on mucous membranes to that of the carbonate producing ulcerations on these surfaces. It is also a powerful cardiac stimulant. Mucosal disease may call for its use; also respiratory conditions showing severe involvement of the lungs. There is usually an excess of mucus with moist cough when this remedy is indicated.

Angustura Vera. N.O. Rutaceae.
Trituration of tree bark.

Bones and muscles come prominently into consideration when this plant is specified. Stiffness and limb pains of varying degree are prominent along with exostosis. Mild paralysis of legs has been noted. The action on bones may lead on to caries with possible fractures developing.

Anthracinum.
The Ø is prepared from affected tissue or culture dissolved in alcohol.

This nosode is indicated in the treatment of eruptive skin diseases which are characterised by boil-like swellings. Cellular tissue becomes indurated and swelling of associated lymph glands takes place. The characteristic lesion assumes the form of a hard swelling with a necrotic centre and surrounded by a blackened rim. It has proved useful in the treatment of septic bites.

Antimonium Arsenicosum. Arsenate of Antimony.
Potencies are prepared from trituration of the dried salt dissolved in distilled water or alcohol.

This salt possesses a selective action on the lungs especially the upper left area and is used mainly in the treatment of emphysema and long-standing pneumonias. Coughing, if present, is worse on eating and the animal prefers to stand rather than lie down.

Antimonium Crudum. Sulphide of Antimony.
Potencies prepared from trituration of the dried salt.

This substance exerts a strong influence on the stomach and skin producing conditions which are aggravated by heat. Any vesicular skin condition should be influenced favourably.

Antimonium Tartaricum. Tartar Emetic.
Trituration of the dried salt is the source of potencies.

Respiratory symptoms predominate with this drug, affections being accompanied by the production of excess mucus, although expectoration is difficult. The main action being on the respiratory system, we should expect this remedy to be beneficial in conditions such as broncho-pneumonia and pulmonary oedema. Ailments requiring this remedy frequently show an accompanying drowsiness and lack of thirst. In pneumonic states the edges of the eyes may be covered with mucus.

Apis Mellifica. Bee Venom.
The Ø is prepared from the entire insect and also from the venom diluted with alcohol.

The poison of the bee acts on cellular tissue causing oedema and swelling. The production of oedema anywhere in the system may lead to a variety of acute and chronic conditions. Considering the well documented evidence of its sphere of action affecting all tissues and mucous membranes, we should consider this remedy in conditions showing oedematous swellings. Synovial swellings of joints may respond to its use. Respiratory conditions showing an excess of pulmonary fluid or oedema, have been treated successfully with this remedy, while it has also been used to good effect in the treatment of cystic ovaries. All ailments are aggravated by heat and are thirstless.

Apocynum Cannabinum. Indian Hemp. N.O Apocynaceae.
Infusions of the fresh plant.

This substance produces disturbance of gastric function along with affection of heart muscle leading to a slowing of its action. There is also a marked action on the uro-genital system producing diuresis and uterine bleeding. The patient requiring this remedy may present symptoms of drowsiness or stupor. Upper respiratory symptoms are common e.g. nasal secretions of yellowish mucus.

Apomorphinum.
This is one of the alkaloids of morphine and has a profound action on the vomiting centre of the brain producing several emissis preceded by increased secretion of saliva and mucous. Pupils become dilated. It is used in veterinary practice to produce complete emptying of stomach contents after suspected poisoning or ingestion of foreign matter, and homoeopathically to control prolonged and severe vomiting.

Argentum Nitricum. Silver Nitrate.
This remedy is prepared by trituration of the salt and subsequent dissolving in alcohol or distilled water.

It produces incoordination of movement causing trembling in various parts. It has an irritant effect on mucous membranes producing a free-flowing muco-purulent discharge. Red blood cells are affected, anaemia being caused by their destruction. Its sphere of action makes it a useful remedy in eye conditions.

Arnica Montana. Leopard's Bane. N.O. Compositae.
The Ø is prepared from the whole fresh plant.

The action of this plant upon the system is practically synonymous with a state resulting from injuries or blows. It is known as the 'Fall Herb' and is used mainly for wounds and injuries where the skin remains unbroken. It has a marked affinity with blood-vessels leading to dilation, stasis and increased permeability. Thus various types of haemorrhage can occur. It reduces shock when given in potency and should be given routinely before and after surgical interference when it will also help control bleeding. Given after parturition it will hasten recovery of bruised tissue, while given during pregnancy at regular intervals, it will help promote normal easy parturition.

Arsenicum Album. Arsenic Trioxide.
This remedy is prepared by trituration and subsequent dilution.

It is a deep acting remedy and acts on every tissue of the body and its characteristic and definite symptoms make its use certain in many ailments. Discharges are acrid and burning and symptoms are relieved by heat. It is of use in many skin conditions associated with dryness, scaliness and itching. It could also have a role to play in some forms of pneumonia when the patient may show a desire for small quantities of water and symptoms becoming worse towards midnight.

Arsenicum Iodatum. Iodide of Arsenic.
Potencies are prepared from the triturated salt dissolved in distilled water.

When discharges are persistently irritating and corrosive, this remedy may prove more beneficial than Arsen. alb. The mucous membranes become red, swollen and oedematous, especially in the respiratory sphere. This remedy is frequently called for in bronchial and pneumonic conditions which are at the convalescent stage or in those ailments which have not responded satisfactorily to seemingly indicated remedies.

Atropinum. An Alkaloid of Belladonna.
This alkaloid produces some of the effects of Belladonna itself but acts more particularly on the eyes causing dilation of pupils and mucous membranes generally which become extremely dry. It could be indicated where overall symptoms of Belladonna are not well-defined.

Baptisia Tinctoria. Wild Indigo. N.O. Leguminosae.
The Ø is prepared from fresh root and bark.

The symptoms produced by this plant relate mainly to septicaemic conditions producing prostration and weakness. Low grade fevers and great muscular lethargy are present in the symptomatology. All secretions and discharges are very offensive. Profuse salivation occurs together with ulceration of gums which become discoloured. Tonsils and throat are dark red and stools tend to be dysenteric. It should be remembered as a possibly useful remedy in some forms of feline enteritis when other symptoms agree.

Baryta Carbonica. Barium Carbonate.
Potencies are prepared from trituration of the salt dissolved in distilled water.

The action of this salt produces symptoms and conditions more usually seen in old and very young subjects and should be remembered as a useful remedy for certain conditions affecting the respiratory system especially.

Baryta Muriatica. Barium Chloride.
Solution of salt in distilled water.

This salt produces periodic attacks of convulsions with spastic involvement of limbs. Ear discharges appear which are offensive and the parotid salivary glands become swollen. Induration of abdominal glands develop including the pancreas. It is indicated in many instances of ear canker and also in animals which show a tendency to develop glandular swellings along with the characteristic involvement of the nervous system.

Belladonna. Deadly Nightshade. N.O. Solanaceae.
The Ø is prepared from the whole plant at flowering.

This plant produces a profound action on every part of the central nervous system causing a state of excitement and active congestion. The effect also on the skin, glands and vascular system is constant and specific. One of the main guiding symptoms in prescribing is the presence of a full bounding pulse in any feverish condition which may or may not accompany excitable states. Another guiding symptom is dilation of pupils.

Bellis Perennis. Daisy. N.O. Compositae.
The Ø is prepared from the whole fresh plant.

The main action of this little flower is on the muscular tissues of blood vessels producing a state of venous congestion. Systemic muscles become heavy leading to a halting type of gait suggestive of pain. This is a useful remedy to aid recovery of tissues injured during cutting or after operation. Sprains and bruises in general come within its sphere of action and it should be kept in mind as an adjunct remedy along with

Arnica. Given post-partum it will hasten resolution of bruised tissue and enable the pelvic area to recover tone in a very short time.

Benzoicum Acidum. Benzoic Acid.
Potencies are prepared from gum benzoin which is triturated and dissolved in alcohol.

The most outstanding feature of this remedy relates to the urinary system producing changes in the colour and odour of the urine, which becomes dark red and aromatic with uric acid deposits. It may have a place in the treatment of some kidney and bladder conditions.

Berberis Vulgaris. Barberry. N.O. Berberidaceae.
The Ø is prepared from the bark of the root.

This shrub of wide distribution has an affinity with most tissues. Symptoms which it produces are liable to alternate violently, e.g. feverish conditions with thirst can quickly give way to prostration without any desire for water. It acts forcibly on the venous system producing especially pelvic engorgements. The chief ailments which come within its sphere of action are those connected with liver and kidney leading to catarrhal inflammation of bile ducts and kidney pelvis. Jaundice frequently attends such conditions. Haematuria and cystitis may occur. In all these conditions there is an accompanying sacral weakness and tenderness over the loins.

Beryllium. The Metal.
Trituration and subsequent dissolving in alcohol produces the tincture from which the potencies are prepared.

This remedy is used mainly in respiratory conditions where the leading symptom is difficult breathing on slight exertion and which is out of proportion to clinical findings. Coughing and emphysema are usually present. This is a useful remedy in virus pneumonia, both acute and chronic forms, where symptoms are few while the animal is resting, but become pronounced on movement. It is a deep acting remedy and should not be used below 30c potency.

Borax. Sodium Biborate.
Potencies are prepared from trituration of the salt dissolved in distilled water.

This salt produces gastro-intestinal irritation with mouth symptoms of salivation and ulceration. With most complaints there is fear of downward motion. The specific action of this substance on the epithelium of the mouth, tongue and buccal mucosa determines its use as a remedy which will control such conditions as vesicular stomatitis and allied diseases, e.g. mucosal disease.

Bothrops Lanceolatus. Yellow Viper.
Potencies are prepared from solution of the venom in glycerine.

This poison is associated with haemorrhages and subsequent rapid coagulation of blood. Septic involvement takes place as a rule and this is, therefore, a useful remedy in septic states showing haemorrhagic tendencies. Gangrenous conditions of the skin may respond to it.

Bromium. Bromine. The Element.
Potencies are prepared from solutions in distilled water.

Bromine is found in combinations with iodine in the ash when seaweed is burned, and also in sea water. It acts chiefly on the mucous membrane of the respiratory tract, especially the upper trachea causing laryngeal spasm. This is a useful remedy for croup-like cough accompanied by rattling of mucus. Its indication in respiratory ailments is related to symptoms being aggravated on inspiration. It may be of use also in those conditions which arise from over-exposure to heat.

Bryonia Alba. White Bryony. Wild Hop. N.O. Cucurbitaceae.
The Ø is prepared from the root before flowering takes place.

This important plant produces a glucoside which is capable of bringing on severe purgation. The plant itself exerts its main action on epithelial tissues and serous and synovial membranes. Some mucous surfaces are also affected producing an inflammatory response resulting in a fibrinous or serous exudate. This in turn leads to dryness of the affected tissue with later effusions into synovial cavities. Movement of the parts is interfered with and this leads to one of the main indications for its use, viz. all symptoms are worse from movement, the animal preferring to lie still. Pressure over affected areas relieves symptoms. This remedy may be extremely useful in treating the many respiratory conditions met with, especially pleurisy where the above symptom picture is seen.

Bufo. The Toad. N.O. Buforidae. Solution of Poison.
This remedy is used in states of cerebral excitement sometimes severe enough to precipitate epilepsy. Dropsical states also develop. Has also been used in cases of exaggerated sexual impulses especially in the male.

Cactus Grandiflorus. Night-Blooming Cereus. N.O. Cactaceae.
The Ø is prepared from young stems and flowers.
  The active principle of this plant acts on circular muscle fibres and has a marked affinity for the cardio-vascular system. It is mainly confined to the treatment of valvular disease, but it may also be of service in some conditions showing a haemorrhagic tendency.

Calcarea Carbonica. Carbonate of Lime.
Trituration of the salt in alcohol or weak acid produces the solution from which potencies are prepared. The crude substance is found in the middle layer of the oyster shell.
  This calcareous substance produces a lack of tone and muscular weakness with muscle spasm affecting both voluntary and involuntary muscles. Calcium is excreted quickly from the system and the intake of calcium salts does not ensure against conditions which may need the element prepared in the homoeopathic manner. Calc. carb. is a strong constitutional remedy causing impaired nutrition, and animals which need potentised calcium show a tendency to eat strange objects. It is of value in the treatment of skeletal disorders of young animals and in the older animal suffering from osteomalacia.

Calcarea Fluorica. Fluorspar. Fluoride of Lime.
Potencies are prepared from trituration of the salt with subsequent dilution in distilled water.
  Crystals of this substance are found in the Haversian canals of bone. This increases the hardness, but in excess produces brittleness. It also occurs in tooth enamel and in the epidermis of the skin. Affinity with all these tissues may lead to the establishment of exostoses and glandular enlargements. It is in addition a powerful vascular remedy. The special sphere of action of this remedy lies in its relation to bone lesions especially exostoses.

Calcarea Iodata. Iodide of Lime.
Solution of salt in distilled water.
  This remedy is used in cases of hardening of tissue, especially glands and tonsils. The thyroid gland is also affected and occasionally the thymus as well.

Calcarea Phosphorica. Phosphate of Lime.
Potencies are prepared from trituration and subsequent dilution, from adding dilute phosphoric acid to lime water.
  This salt has an affinity with tissues which are concerned with growth and the repair of cells. Assimilation may be difficult because of impaired nutrition and delayed development. Brittleness of bone is a common feature. This is a remedy of special value in the treatment of musculo-skeletal disorders of young animals.

Calc. Renalis Phosph and Calc. Renalis Uric.
These two salts are indicated in cases of lithiasis due to the presence of stones of the respective substances. They aid the action of remedies such as Berberis and Hydrangea and Thlaspi and can be used along with them.

Calendula Officinalis. Marigold. N.O. Compositae.
The Ø is prepared from leaves and flowers.
  Applied locally to open wounds and indolent ulcers this remedy will be found to be one of the most reliable healing agents we have. It will rapidly bring about resolution of tissue promoting healthy granulation. It should be used as a 1/10 dilution in warm water. It is helpful in treating contused wounds of the eyes and it can be combined with Hypericum when treating open wounds involving damage to nerves.

Calici Virus.
The potentised virus can be used either by itself or combined with other viruses in the treatment of gingivitis and respiratory conditions where it is thought that the disease is implicated.

Camphora. Camphor. N.O. Lauraceae.
Potencies are prepared from a solution of the gum in rectified spirit.

20

This substance produces a state of collapse with weakness and failing pulse. There is icy coldness of the entire body. It has a marked relationship to muscles and fasciae. Certain forms of scour will benefit from this remedy, viz. those forms accompanied by collapse and extreme coldness of body surfaces. Any form of enteritis showing exhaustion and collapse may require this remedy. It may be needed in disease caused by salmonella species.

Cannabis Sativa. American Hemp. N.O. Cannabinaceae.
The Ø is prepared from the flowering tops of the plant. This plant affects particularly the urinary, sexual and respiratory systems, conditions being accompanied by great fatigue. There is a tendency to pneumonia, pericarditis and retention of urine; this may lead to cystitis and a mucoid blood-stained urine.

Cantharis. Spanish Fly.
The Ø is prepared by trituration of the insect with subsequent dilution in alcohol.
The poisonous substances contained in this insect attack particularly the urinary and sexual organs setting up violent inflammation. The skin is also markedly affected, a severe vesicular rash developing with intense itching. This is a valuable remedy in nephritis and cystitis typified by frequent attempts at urination, the urine itself containing blood as a rule. It may be indicated in certain post-partum inflammations and burning vesicular eczemas.

Carbo Vegetabilis. Vegetable Charcoal.
Potencies are prepared by trituration and subsequent dilution in alcohol.
Various tissues of the body have a marked affinity with this substance. The circulatory system is particularly affected leading to lack of oxygenation with a corresponding increase of carbon dioxide in the blood and tissues. This in turn leads to a lack of resistance to infections and to haemorrhages of dark blood which does not readily coagulate. Coldness of the body surface supervenes. When potentised this is a very useful remedy in all cases of collapse. Pulmonary congestions will benefit and it restores warmth and strength in cases of circulatory weakness. It acts more on the venous than on the arterial circulation.

21

Carduus Marianus. St. Mary's Thistle. N.O. Compositae.
Trituration of seeds dissolved in spirits.

This remedy is indicated in disorders arising from inefficiency of liver function. The action of the liver indicates its main use in veterinary practice. Cirrhotic conditions with accompanying dropsy respond well.

Caulophyllum. Blue Cohosh. N.O. Berberidaceae.
The Ø is prepared from trituration of the root dissolved in alcohol.

This plant produces pathological states related to the female genital system. Extraordinary rigidity of the *os uteri* is set up leading to difficulties at parturition. Early abortions may occur due to uterine debility. These may be accompanied by fever and thirst. There is a tendency to retention of afterbirth with possible bleeding from the uterus. In potentised form this remedy will revive labour pains and could be used as an alternative to pituitrin injections once the os is open. It will be found useful in ringwomb and also in cases of uterine twist or displacement. In these cases it should be given frequently for three or four doses, e.g. hourly intervals. In animals which have had previous miscarriages it will help in establishing a normal pregnancy while post-partum it is one of the remedies to be considered for retained afterbirth.

Causticum. Potassium Hydroxide.
This substance is prepared by the distillation of a mixture of equal parts of slaked lime and potassium bisulphate.

The main affinity is with the neuro-muscular system producing weakness and paresis of both types of muscle. Symptoms are aggravated by going from a cold atmosphere to a warm one. It may be of use in bronchitic conditions of older animals and in those which develop small sessile warts. It appears to have an antidotal effect in cases of lead poisoning and could be used in this connection as an adjunct to versenate injections.

Ceanothus Americanus. New Jersey Tea. N.O. Rhamnaceae.
Tincture of fresh leaves.

Splenic conditions in general come within the range of this remedy. Tenderness of the spleen may be evident. In the female whitish vaginal discharges may arise. Chiefly used for conditions where it is thought that the spleen is involved.

Chelidonium. Greater Celandine. N.O. Papaveraceae.
The Ø is prepared from the whole plant, fresh at the time of flowering.
   A specific action on the liver is produced by this plant. There is general lethargy and indisposition. The tongue is usually coated a dirty yellow and signs of jaundice may be seen in other visible mucous membranes. The liver is constantly upset with the production of clay-coloured stools. Because of its marked hepatic action it should be remembered when dealing with disturbances associated with a sluggish liver action. It may be of use in photosensitisation if signs of jaundice occur.

Chimaphilla Umbellata. Ground Holly. N.O. Ericaceae.
The Ø is prepared from the fresh plant.
   The active principle of this plant produces a marked action on the kidneys and genital system of both sexes. In the eyes cataracts may develop. The urine is mucoid and blood-stained. Enlargement of prostate gland may develop while in the female mammary tumours and atrophy have both been recorded.

Chininum Sulphuricum. Sulphate of Quinine.
Trituration of salt dissolved in alcohol.
   This salt closely resembles the action of China and should be remembered as a useful remedy in cases of debility due to loss of essential fluids. It affects the ear producing pain over the area and excessive secretion of wax. Conditions calling for its use tend to recur after apparent or real remissions. Septic conditions of the cat, following bites or injuries, respond well and thereby reduce the likelihood of future tissue involvement of a septic nature.

Chionanthus Virginica. Fringe Tree.
Tincture of bark.
   This remedy is indicated in sluggish states of the liver including early cases of cirrhosis, accompanying a generalised loss of condition and in extreme cases emaciation. The stools produced are clay-coloured and there may be jaundice and high-coloured urine.

Chlamydia
This potentised nosode is used to prevent chlamydial infection in young cats (see main text) and also in the treatment of kittens showing the typical symptoms of gummy eyes and other manifestations.

Cinchona Officinalis. China Officinalis. Peruvian Bark. N.O. Rubiaceae.
The Ø is prepared from the dried bark dissolved in alcohol.

This plant is commonly referred to as 'China' and is the source of quinine. Large doses tend to produce toxic changes, e.g. nervous sensitivity, impaired leucocyte formation, haemorrhages, fever and diarrhoea. Weakness ensues from loss of body fluids. This remedy should be considered when an animal is suffering from debility or exhaustion after fluid loss, e.g. severe diarrhoea or haemorrhage. It is seldom indicated in the earlier stages of acute disease.

Cinnabaris. Mercuric Sulphide.
Trituration of salt dissolved in alcohol.

The action of this substance relates mainly to the genito-urinary sphere where conditions such as albuminuria and balanitis tend to occur. Warts develop in the inguinal area. Eye conditions are also common such as blepharitis and ophthalmia with purulent discharge. Sometimes the ear is affected producing a dry itching condition with scurf around the pinna. Chiefly used in practice where other mercurial remedies have given less than satisfactory results.

Cicuta Virosa. Water Hemlock. N.O. Umbelliferae.
The Ø is prepared from the fresh root at the time of flowering.

The central nervous system is principally affected by this plant, spasmodic affections occurring. A characteristic feature is the head and neck twisted to one side accompanied by violence of one kind or another. Aggravation occurs from jarring or sudden movement. The general balance becomes upset and there is a tendency to fall to one side while the head and spine bend backwards. Various conditions of the brain and spinal cord may benefit from this remedy, e.g. cerebro-cortical necrosis, showing the typical lateral deviation of neck.

Cineraria Maritima. Dusty Miller. N.O. Compositae.
The Ø is prepared from the whole fresh plant.

The active principle is used mainly as an external application in eye conditions. The Ø should be diluted 1/10.

Cobaltum. The Metal. Cobaltum Chloridum. The Salt.
Both these remedies are used mainly in the 30c potency in the treatment of cobalt deficiency and give good results over a period of a few weeks.

Cocculus. Indian Cockle. N.O. Menispermacrae.
The Ø is prepared from powdered seeds which contain an alkaloid pectoxin.

The active principle produces spasmodic and paretic affections deriving from the CNS (Cerebrum), not the spinal cord. There is a strong tendency to vomit due to the action on the vomiting centre which appears to be dependent on movement. Mainly used in travel sickness where symptoms agree.

Coccus Cacti. Cochineal.
The Ø is prepared from the dried bodies of the female insects.

This substance has an affinity for mucous membranes producing catarrhal inflammation. Viscid mucus accumulates in the air passages leading to difficulty in expectoration and spasmodic coughing. Dysuria is common, the urine being scanty and leaving a reddish deposit on standing. It is mainly used in affections of the respiratory and urinary systems.

Colchicum Autumnale. Meadow Saffron. N.O. Liliaceae.
The Ø is prepared from the bulb.

This plant affects muscular tissues, periosteum and synovial membranes of joints. It possesses also an anti-allergic and anti-inflammatory action which interferes with the natural recuperative powers of the body. Illnesses which may require this remedy are usually acute and severe, accompanied frequently by effusions in the small joints. Autumnal diarrhoea and dysentery also may be helped, the latter accompanied by tympany and tenesmus. One of its guiding

25

symptoms is aversion to food, while complaints requiring it are generally worse from movement.

Colocynthis. Bitter Cucumber. N.O. Cucurbitaceae.
The Ø is prepared from the fruit and contains a glucoside — colocynthin.

This plant is purgative and causes violent inflammatory lesions of the gastro-intestinal tract. Both onset of and relief from symptoms are abrupt. Diarrhoea is yellowish and forcibly expelled. Relief is obtained by movement while aggravation occurs after eating or drinking.

Condurango. Condor Plant.
The Ø is prepared from bark in tincture.

This plant produces a glucoside condurangin which affects the nervous system causing an exaggerated gait. It can act constitutionally in promoting the general well-being of the patient. More specifically there is an action on epithelial tissue causing hardening which may lead on to tumour formation. A guiding symptom is said to be cracks at the corners of the mouth. Chiefly used as a remedy to combat incipient cancerous states especially those in the abdomen.

Conium Maculatum. Hemlock. N.O. Umbelliferae.
The Ø is prepared from the fresh plant.

The alkaloid of this plant produces a paralytic action on nerve ganglia, especially the motor nerve endings. This leads to stiffness and a paralysis which tends to travel forward or upward. This remedy is of importance in treating paraplegic conditions and any weakness of hind limbs.

Convallaria Majalis. Lily of the Valley. N.O. Liliaceae.
The Ø is prepared from the fresh plant.

The active principle has the power to increase the quality of the heart's action and this determines its main use as a remedy in congestive heart conditions. It has little action on the heart muscle and is used mainly in valvular disease.

Copaiva. Balsam of Peru. N.O. Leguminosae.
The Ø is prepared from the balsam.

26

This substance produces a marked action on mucous membranes, especially those of the urinary and respiratory tracts causing a catarrhal inflammation. This action makes the remedy useful in the treatment of urethritis and cystitis. Pyelonephritis is one of the commoner conditions which could be helped.

Cortisone
The potentised steroid is used in practice to combat the effects of the over prescribing of the crude substance where very often a single dose of the 200c potency will suffice along with clearing remedies such as *Nux Vomica* and *Thuja*. In lower potency e.g. 12c – 30c it helps in certain skin conditions where dryness and redness predominate along with excessive itching.

Crataegus. Hawthorn. N.O. Rosaceae.
The Ø is prepared from the ripe fruit.
   The active principle produces a fall in blood pressure and brings on dyspnoea. It acts on the heart muscle causing an incease in the number and quality of contractions. The specific action on the heart muscle makes this a particularly useful remedy in the treatment of arrhythmic heart conditions.

Crotalus Horridus. Rattlesnake.
The Ø is prepared from trituration of the venom with lactose and subsequent dilution in glycerine.
   This venom produces sepsis, haemorrhages and jaundice with decomposition of blood. The marked action of this poison on the vascular system makes it a valuable remedy in the treatment of many low-grade septic states with circulatory involvement, e.g. puerperal fever and wound infections. Septic conditions are accompanied by oozing of blood from any body orifice and are usually attended by jaundice. It should help in conditions such as adder-bite.

Croton Tiglium. Croton Oil Seeds. N.O. Euphorbiaceae.
The Ø is prepared from the oil obtained from the seeds.
   This oil produces violent diarrhoea and skin eruptions causing inflammation with a tendency to vesicle formation. This is one of the

many useful remedies for controlling diarrhoea. This is usually accompanied by great urging, the stool being watery.

Cryptococcus
This potentised nosode is used as for chlamydia and calici and can be combined with them if need be in multiple infections.

Cubeba Officinalis. Cubebs. N.O. Piperaceae.
The Ø is prepared from the dried unripe fruit.
 The active principle acts on mucous membranes producing a catarrhal inflammation. Those of the uro-genital tract are particularly affected, the urine becoming cloudy and albuminous.

Cuprum Aceticum. Copper Acetate.
Potencies are prepared from a solution in distilled water.
 This salt produces cramping of muscles, spasms and paralytic conditions.

Cuprum Metallicum. Metallic Copper.
The Ø is prepared from trituration of the metal.
 The symptoms produced by this metal are characterised by violence including paroxysms of cramping pains which follow no particular pattern. Muscles become contracted and show twitchings. In the central nervous system fits and convulsions occur and may take an epileptiform nature. The head is drawn to one side.

Curare. Woorara. Arrow Poison.
The Ø is prepared from dilutions in alcohol.
 This poison produces muscular paralysis without impairing sensation or consciousness. Reflex action is diminished and a state of motor paralysis sets in. It decreases the output of adrenaline and brings about a state of nervous debility.

Damiana
The active principle of this plant has an affinity for the sexual system and is used mainly to promote libido in the male animal where sexual drive is weak. The action and results are variable but it is a remedy to keep in mind in this connection.

Digitalis Purpurea. Foxglove. N.O. Scrophulariaceae.
The Ø is prepared from the leaves.

The active principle of the foxglove causes marked slowness of the heart's action, the pulse being weak and irregular. This is a commonly used remedy in heart conditions helping to regulate the beat and producing a stable pulse. By increasing the output of the heart when used in low potencies it aids valvular function. This in turn increases the output of urine and helps reduce oedema.

Drosera Rotundifolia. Sundew. N.O. Droseraceae.
The Ø is prepared from the fresh plant.

The lymphatic and pleural systems together with synovial membranes are all affected by this plant. The laryngeal area is also subject to inflammatory processes, any timulus producing a hypersensitive reaction.

Dulcamara. Woody Nightshade. N.O. Solanaceae.
The Ø is prepared from the green stems and leaves before flowering.

This plant belongs to the same family as Belladonna, Hyoscyamus and Stramonium. Tissue affinities are with mucous membranes, glands and kidneys, producing inflammatory changes and interstitial haemorrhages. This remedy may benefit those conditions which arise as a result of exposure to wet and cold, especially when damp evenings follow a warm day. Such conditions commonly occur in autumn and diarrhoea occurring then may benefit. It has proved useful in the treatment of ringworm and could have a beneficial action on large fleshy warts.

Echinacea Angustifolia. Rudbeckia. N.O. Compositae.
The Ø is prepared from the whole plant.

Acute toxaemias with septic involvement of various tissues come within the sphere of action of this plant. It is a valuable remedy in the treatment of post-partum puerperal conditions where sepsis is evident. Generalised septic states having their origin in infected bites or stings will also benefit. This remedy acts best in low decimal potencies.

E. coli
This organism is found in the bowel and plays an essential role in the digestive process. As a remedy the nosode is used in bowel conditions

where scouring develops after stress in the young animal or where the balance of the bowel flora has been interfered with.

Eel Serum.
The Ø is prepared from dried serum or solution in distilled water.

The serum of the eel produces an action on the blood equivalent to toxaemia. It affects the kidney particularly with secondary effects on the liver. Renal deposits are found in the urine along with haemoglobin. Threatened anaemic states develop. The cardiac system is also affected, sudden fainting spells being common.

Epigea Repens. Trailing Arbutus. N.O. Ericaceae.
The Ø is prepared from tincture of fresh leaves.

The main action of this remedy is on the urinary system where it produces a state of strangury with the production of renal calculi. It should be remembered in this connection as a useful remedy in cystitis of both male and female cats and in the treatment of urethral and bladder stones.

Euphrasia Officinalis. Eyebright. N.O. Scrophulariaceae.
The Ø is prepared from the whole plant.

The active principle acts mainly on the conjunctival mucous membrane producing lachrymation. The cornea is also affected, opacities being common. This is one of the most useful remedies in the treatment of a variety of eye conditions, principally conjunctivitis and corneal ulcerations. Internal treatment should be supplemented by its use externally as a lotion diluted 1/10.

F.V.R. Nosode.
This is the potentised virus prepared from a case of feline viral rhinotracheitis. It can be used in both the prophylactic and therapeutic manner, and in the former combined with other viral nosodes.

Ferrum Iodatum. Iodide of Iron.
Potencies are prepared from trituration of crystals subsequently dissolved in alcohol.

This salt is chiefly of interest as a remedy for iron deficiency associated with respiratory distress, mucous discharges containing blood being present. Metallic iron (Ferrum Metallicum) and chloride of iron (Ferrum Muriaticum) are also used in the treatment of iron deficiency, the former particularly for younger animals and the latter more indicated when heart symptoms such as weak thready pulse are present.

Ferrum Phosphoricum. Ferric Phosphate.
Potencies are prepared from a solution in distilled water.
Febrile conditions in general are associated with this salt. It is frequently used in the early stages of inflammatory conditions which develop less rapidly than those calling for Aconitum. Throat involvement is often the key to its selection. Pulmonary congestions may call for its use if haemorrhages are also present.

Ficus Religiosa. Pakur. N.O. Moraceae.
The Ø is prepared from fresh leaves in alcohol.
Haemorrhages of various kinds are associated with the toxic effects of this plant. Any condition which produces bleeding of a bright red character may indicate the need for this remedy, but generally respiratory rather than digestive upsets determine its use.

Fluoricum Acidum. Hydrofluoric Acid.
Potencies are prepared by distilling calcium fluoride with sulphuric acid.
It has an action on most tissues producing deep-seated ulcers and lesions of a destructive nature. It has been used successfully in the treatment of ulcerative conditions of the mouth and throat. Any necrotic condition of bone is likely to benefit.

Folliculinum.
This is one of the ovarian hormones which has a beneficial action on the skin. Used mainly in practice in cases of miliary eczema and alopecia of both sexes. It can also be used in the treatment of eczemas of non-hormonal origin where the typical purply rashes predominate.

Formica. Formic Acid. The Ant. N.O. Hymenoptera.
Tincture made from live ants. This acid produces rheumatic-like pains along with deposits in the small joints. Occasionally in severe cases the spinal cord may be affected giving rise to a state of temporary paralysis.

It is chiefly used in veterinary practice as an anti-arthritis remedy especially affecting carpal and tarsal areas.

Gaertner-Bach.
Marked emaciation or malnutrition is associated with this nosode. Chronic gastro-enteritis occurs and there is a tendency for the animal to become infested with worms. There is an inability to digest fat. Chiefly used in the young animal showing malnutrition associated with other digestive problems.

Gelsemium Sempervirens. Yellow Jasmine. N.O. Loganiaceae.
The Ø is prepared from the bark of the root.
The affinity of this plant is with the nervous system producing varying degrees of motor paralysis. This remedy has proved helpful as a supportive measure in hypomagnesaemia, aiding restoration of normal movement. Single paralysis of different nerves, e.g. the radial may also benefit. Conditions which call for its use are usually attended by weakness and muscle tremors.

Glonoinum. Nitro-Glycerine.
Potencies are prepared from dilutions in alcohol.
This substance has an affinity with the brain and circulatory system causing sudden and violent convulsions and also congestion in the arterial system leading to throbbing and pulsations, seen in superficial vessels. It will be found of use in brain conditions arising from over-exposure to heat or the effects of the sun. It may also help the convulsions and allied conditions.

Graphites. Black Lead.
Potencies are prepared from triturations dissolved in alcohol.
This form of carbon has an affinity with skin. Eruptions are common and its action on connective tissue tends to produce fibrotic conditions associated with malnutrition. Loss of hair occurs while purply moist eruptions ooze a sticky discharge. Abrasions develop into ulcers which may suppurate. Favourable sites for eczema are in the bends of joints and behind the ears.

Hamamelis Virginica. Witch Hazel. N.O. Hamamelidaceae.
The Ø is prepared from fresh bark of twigs and roots.

This plant has an affinity with the venous circulation producing congestions and haemorrhages. The action on the veins is one of relaxation, with consequent engorgement. Any condition showing venous engorgement or congestion with passive haemorrhage should show improvement from the use of this remedy.

Hecla Lava. Hecla.
Potencies are prepared from triturition of the volcanic ash. Present in this ash are the substances which accompany lava formation, viz. Alumina, Lime and Silica.

Lymphoid tissue and the skeleton are areas which show the greatest affinity for this substance. The remedy is useful in the treatment of exostoses or tumours of the facial bones and in caries arising from dental disease. It has proved successful in the treatment of conditions affecting the maxillary and mandibular bones. It should help in the treatment of bony tumours generally.

Helleborus Niger. Christmas Rose. N.O. Ranunculaceae.
The Ø is produced from the juice of the fresh root.

The affinity of this plant is with the central nervous system and the alimentary canal. To a lesser extent the kidneys are involved. Vertigo-like movements arise together with convulsions. Vomiting and purging take place, stools being dysenteric. Heart action is slowed.

Hepar Sulphuris Calcareum. Impure Calcium Sulphide.
This substance is prepared by burning crude calcium carbonate with flowers of sulphur. Potencies are then prepared from the triturated ash.

This remedy is associated with suppurative processes producing conditions which are extremely sensitive to touch. It causes catarrhal and purulent inflammation of the mucous membranes of the respiratory and alimentary tracts with involvement of the skin and lymphatic system. This remedy has a wide range of action and should be considered in any suppurative process showing extreme sensitivity to touch indicating acute pain. Low potencies of this remedy promote suppuration while high potencies — 200c and upwards — may abort the purulent process and promote resolution.

Hippozaeninum.
This nosode has been known for a long time having been made from glanders, a notifiable equine disease no longer encountered in Britain. It has a wide range of use in many catarrhal conditions which are characterised by glutinous or honey-coloured discharges, e.g. sinusitis and ozaena with or without ulceration of nasal cartilages. It could be of great benefit in some forms of chronic viral rhinitis.

Hydrangea Arborescons. N.O. Hydrangeaceae.
The Ø is prepared from fresh leaves and young shoots.
   This plant exerts a strong influence on the urinary system, especially on the bladder where it helps dissolve gravel. The prostate gland also comes within its range of action.

Hydrastis Canadensis. Golden Seal. N.O. Ranunculaceae.
The Ø is prepared from the fresh root.
   Mucous membranes are affected by this plant, a catarrhal inflamma tion being established. Secretions generally are thick and yellow. Any catarrhal condition resulting in a muco-purulent discharge will come within the scope of this remedy, e.g. mild forms of metritis or sinusitis.

Hydrocotyle Asiatica. Indian Pennywort. N.O. Umbelliferae.
The Ø is prepared from the whole plant.
   The main difficulty of this plant is with the skin and female genital system. It also has a lesser effect on the action of the liver. Skin conditions showing thickening of epidermis and roughening come within its sphere of action.

Hyoscyamus Niger. Henbane. N.O. Solanaceae.
The Ø is prepared from the fresh plant.
   The active principle disturbs the central nervous system producing symptoms of brain excitement and mania. Conditions which call for its use are not accompanied by inflammation (cf. Belladonna).

Hypericum Perforatum. St. John's Wort. N.O. Hyperiaceae.
The Ø is prepared from the whole fresh plant.
   The active principle is capable of causing sensitivity to light on some skins in the absence of melanin pigment. The main affinity is with the nervous system causing hypersensitivity. Sloughing and necrosis of

skin may take place. This remedy is of prime importance in the treatment of lacerated wounds where nerve endings are damaged. In spinal injuries, especially of the coccygeal area, it gives good results. The specific action on nerves suggests its use in tetanus where, given early after injury, it helps prevent the spread of toxin. It can be used externally for lacerated wounds along with Calendula, both in a strength of 1/10. It has been found useful in the treatment of photosensitisation and similar allergies.

Iodium. Iodine. The Element.
Potencies are prepared from the tincture prepared by dissolving the element in alcohol. A 1% tincture is the strength used in preparation.

In large doses — iodism — sinuses and eyes are at first involved leading to conjunctivitis and bronchitis. Iodine has a special affinity with the thyroid gland. Weakness and atrophy of muscles may follow excessive intake. The skin becomes dry and withered looking and the appetite becomes voracious. Conditions which show a characteristic oppositeness of symptoms, e.g. tissue hyperplasia or atrophy may need this remedy. It may be of use in ovarian dysfunction when the ovaries appear small and shrunken on rectal examination. It is a useful gland remedy and its specific relation to the thyroid should not be forgotten.

Ipecacuanha. N.O. Rubiaceae.
The Ø is prepared from the dried root. Emetine, an alkaloid is its principal constituent.

This plant is associated with haemorrhages and has found a use in the treatment of post-partum bleeding where the blood comes in gushes. Some forms of diarrhoea may also benefit, particularly those showing tenesmus with greenish stools.

Iris Versicolour. Blue Flag. N.O. Iridaceae.
The Ø is prepared from the fresh root.

This plant produces an action on various glands, principally the salivary, intestinal pancreas and thyroid. It has a reputation also for aiding the secretion of bile. Due to its action on the thyroid gland swelling of the throat may occur. The remedy is chiefly used in veterinary practice in the treatment of disorders of the pancreas where it has given consistently good results.

Kali Arsenicum. Fowler's Solution. Potassium Arsenite.
Dilutions of this salt provide the Ø.
   The main action is exerted on the skin, a dry scaly eczema with itching being established. It is a good general skin remedy.

Kali Bichromicum. Potassium Bichromate.
Potencies are prepared from a solution in distilled water.
   This salt acts on the mucous membranes of the stomach, intestines and respiratory tract with lesser involvement of other organs. Feverish states are absent. The action on the mucous membranes produces a catarrhal discharge of a tough stringy character with a yellow colour. This particular type of discharge is a strong guiding symptom for its use. It could be used in broncho-pneumonia, sinusitis and pyelo-nephritis.

Kali Carbonicum. Potassium Carbonate.
Potencies are prepared from a solution in distilled water.
   This salt is found in all plants and in the soil, the colloid material of cells containing potassium.
   It produces a generalised weakness which is common to other potassium salts. Feverish states are absent. It could be a useful convalescent remedy.

Kali Chloricum. Potassium Chlorate.
Potencies are prepared from a solution in distilled water.
   The urinary organs are chiefly affected, producing a blood-stained and albuminous urine with a high phosphate content.

Kali Hydriodicum. Potassium Iodide.
Potencies are prepared from triturations dissolved in alcohol.
   This important drug produces an acrid watery discharge from the eyes and also acts on fibrous and connective tissue. Glandular swellings also appear. This is a widely used remedy in various conditions showing the typical eye and respiratory symptoms.

Kreosotum. Beechwood Kreosote.
The Ø is prepared from solution in rectified spirit.

This substance produces haemorrhages from small wounds with burning discharges and ulcerations. It also causes rapid decomposition of body fluids. Blepharitis occurs with a tendency to gangrene of the skin, while in the female dark blood appears from the uterus. This substance has been successfully used in threatened gangrenous states showing the typical early stages of spongy bleeding and ulceration.

Lachesis. Bushmaster. Surucucu Snake.
Trituration of venom dissolved in alcohol is the source of the solution which yields the potencies.

This venom produces decomposition of blood rendering it more fluid. There is a strong tendency to haemorrhage and sepsis with profound prostration. This is a useful remedy for Adder bites helping to prevent septic complications and reducing swelling. It is particularly valuable if the throat develops inflammation causing left-sided swelling which may involve the parotid gland. Where haemorrhage takes place the blood is dark and does not clot readily while the skin surrounding any lesion assumes a purplish appearance.

Lathyrus Sativus. Chick Pea. N.O. Leguminosae.
The Ø is prepared from the flower and the pods.

This plant affects the anterior columns of the spinal cord producing paralysis of the lower extremities. Nerve power generally is weakened. It should be considered in recumbent conditions associated with mineral deficiencies and in any state involving nerve weakness leading to local paralysis.

Ledum Palustre. Marsh Tea. Wild Rosemary. N.O. Ericaceae.
The Ø is prepared from the whole plant.

The active principle produces tetanus-like symptoms with twitching of muscles. It is one of the main remedies for punctured wounds, especially when the surrounding area becomes cold and discoloured. Insect bites respond well. Also injuries to the eye.

Lemna Minor. Duckweed. N.O. Lemnaceae.
The Ø is prepared from whole fresh plants.

This is a remedy for catarrhal conditions affecting mainly the nasal passages: a muco-purulent nasal discharge develops which is extremely offensive. In the alimentary sphere diarrhoea and flatulence can occur.

Lilium Tigrinum. Tiger Lily. N.O. Liliaceae.
The Ø is prepared from fresh leaves and flowers.

The action is mainly on the pelvic organs producing conditions which arise from uterine or ovarian disturbances. Urine is scanty and frequently passed. An irregular pulse accompanies an increased heart rate. Congestion and blood-stained discharges arise from the uterus and there may be slight prolapse. Indicated in some forms of pyometra where blood is present and also in ovarian disturbances.

Lithium Carbonicum. Lithium Carbonate.
The Ø is prepared from trituration of the dried salt.

This salt produces a chronic arthritic state with a uric acid diathesis. There is difficulty in passing urine which contains mucus and a red sandy deposit. Cystitis develops leading to a dark urine. It is a useful remedy to consider in some forms of arthritis and urinary conditions producing uric acid deposits.

Lobelia Inflata. Indian Tobacco. N.O. Lobeliaceae.
The Ø is prepared from the dried leaves with subsequent dilution in alcohol.

The active principle acts as a vaso-motor stimulant impeding respiration and producing symptoms of inappetance and relaxation of muscles. It is of value in emphysematous conditions and as a general convalescent remedy.

Lycopodium Clavatum. Club Moss. N.O. Lycopodiaceae.
The Ø is prepared from trituration of the spores and dilution in alcohol. The spores are inactive until triturated and potentised.

The active principle acts chiefly on the digestive and renal systems. The respiratory system is also affected, pneumonia being a frequent complication. There is general lack of gastric function and very little food will satisfy. The abdomen becomes bloated with tenderness over the liver. The glycogenic function of the liver is interfered with. This is a very useful remedy in various digestive, urinary and respiratory conditions, a guiding symptom being that complaints frequently show an aggravation in the late afternoon or early evening. Its action on the skin suggests its use in alopecia.

Lycopus Virginicus. Bugle Weed. N.O. Labiatae.
The Ø is prepared from fresh whole plant.

The active principle of this plant reduces blood pressure and causes passive haemorrhages. The main sphere of action which concerns veterinary practice is on the cardiac system where the pulse becomes weak and irregular. The heart's action is increased and is accompanied by difficult breathing and cyanosis. Breathing assumes a wheezy character and may produce a blood-tinged cough.

Magnesia Phosphorica. Phosphate of Magnesium.
Potencies are prepared from trituration of the salt in solution.

This salt acts on muscles producing a cramping effect with spasm.

Malandrinum.
This nosode has been developed from the condition known as grease in the horse after trituration of affected material and discharge. It is used mainly in the treatment of chronic skin eruptions and discharges. In this connection it is worth remembering as a remedy which might help some forms of ear canker.

Melilotus. Sweet Clover. N.O. Leguminosae.
The Ø is prepared from the whole fresh plant.

This plant is associated with profuse haemorrhages. Clover contains a haemolytic agent which prevents clotting of blood after mechanical injuries. It should be remembered as a possibly useful remedy in haematomas and subcutaneous bleeding of unknown origin.

Mercurius. Mercurius Solubilis. Mercury.
Potencies are prepared from triturations and dilutions in alcohol.

This metal affects most organs and tissues producing cellular degeneration with consequent anaemia. Salivation accompanies most complaints and gums become spongy and bleed easily. Diarrhoea is common, stools being slimy and blood-stained. Conditions calling for its use are worse in the period sunset to sunrise.

Mercurius Corrosivus. Mercuric Chloride. Corrosive Sublimate.
Potencies are prepared from triturations and subsequent dilution.

This salt has a somewhat similar action to mercurius, but generally the symptoms produced are more severe. It produces severe tenesmus of the lower bowel leading to dysentery and also has a destructive action on kidney tissue. Discharges from mucous surfaces assume a greenish tinge.

Mercurius Cyanatus. Cyanate of Mercury.
Potencies are prepared from triturations and dilutions.

This particular salt produces an action similar to that associated with bacterial toxins. A haemorrhagic tendency with prostration is a common feature. Ulceration of the mucous membranes of the mouth and throat commonly occur. A greyish membrane surrounds these ulcerated surfaces. The phyaryngeal area is one of the main regions to be affected, redness of the membrane preceding necrosis in the later stages.

Mercurius Dulcis. Calomel. Mercurous Chloride.
Potencies are prepared from triturations and dilution.

This salt has an affinity with the ear and liver especially. Hepatitis with jaundice may result. It is worth considering as a possibly useful remedy in mild forms of cirrhosis.

Mercurius Iodatus Flavus. Yellow Iodide of Mercury.
Potencies are prepared from triturations in dilution.

Mercurous Iodide produces a tendency to glandular induration with attendant coating of the tongue. Sub-maxillary and parotid glands become swollen, more pronounced on the right side. Various swellings of glandular tissue come within the sphere of this remedy, e.g. parotitis and lymphadenitis generally.

Mercurius Iodatus Ruber. Red Iodide of Mercury.
Potencies are prepared from trituration of the salt.

Mercuric Iodide also has a tendency to produce glandular swellings, but in this case the left side of the throat is involved. Stiffness of neck mucles may be a prominent symptom.

Millefolium. Yarrow. N.O. Compositae.
The Ø is prepared from the whole plant.
  Haemorrhages occur from various parts from the action of this plant. The blood is bright red.

Mineral Extract.
This substance has recently been researched and has been shown to have a beneficial effect on certain forms of joint trouble, e.g. arthritis and stiffness especially of the carpal and tarsal areas.

Mixed Grasses.
Some animals show an allergic response to grasses in early spring and summer when excessive itching and skin lesions develop. A combination of various grasses in potency appear to help these conditions and can be combined with other selected remedies.

Morgan-Bach.
Clinical observation has revealed the symptom picture of the bacillus Morgan to cover in general digestive and respiratory conditions with a secondary action on fibrous tissues and skin used mainly in practice to treat inflammatory conditions especially acute eczema combined with appropriate remedies.

Murex Purpurea. Purple Fish.
The Ø is prepared from the dried secretion of the purple gland of one of the Murex species.
  It exerts its action mainly on the female genital system producing irregularities of the oestrus cycle. It has been employed both in anoestrus and for stimulating ovulation, but probably it will give best results in cystic ovary leading to nymphomania.

Muriatic Acid. Hydrochloric Acid.
Potencies are prepared from dilutions, in distilled water.
  This acid produces a blood condition analogous to that associated with septic feverish states of a chronic nature. There is a tendency for ulcers to form. The throat becomes dark red and oedematous while ulceration of lips accompanies swollen gums and neck glands.

Naja Tripudians. Cobra.
Potencies are prepared from trituration of the venom and subsequent dilution in alcohol. Alternatively the Ø may be prepared by dilution of the pure venom.

This poison produces a bulbar paralysis. Haemorrhages are scanty but oedema is marked. The underlying tissues appear dark purple after a bite, blood-stained fluid being present in large quantities. Loss of limb control supervenes. The heart is markedly affected. It could be of use in angio-neurotic oedema.

Natrum Muriaticum. Common Salt. Sodium Chloride.
Potencies are prepared from triturations dissolved in distilled water.

Excessive intake of common salt leads to anaemia, evidenced by dropsy or oedema of various parts. White blood cells are increased while mucous membranes are rendered dry. This is a remedy which is of value in unthrifty conditions arising as a result of anaemia or chronic nephritis.

Natrum Sulphuricum. Sodium Sulphate.
The Ø is prepared from trituration of the salt.

Glauber's Salts (as it is commonly called) produces a state of weakness where the animal has been exposed to damp. The liver is affected and there is a tendency to wart formation. Hepatitis sometimes occurs with jaundice. Flatulent distension and watery diarrhoea supervene. Experience has shown that this remedy has proved to be of great value where there has been a history of head injury leading to a variety of seemingly unrelated conditions.

Nitricum Acidum. Nitric Acid.
Potencies are prepared from a solution in distilled water.

This acid affects particularly body outlets where skin and mucous membranes meet. It produces ulceration and blisters in the mouth and causes offensive discharges. The ulceration may also affect mucous membranes elsewhere and it has been of benefit in some forms of mucosal disease.

Nux Vomica. Poison Nut. N.O. Loganiaeceae.
The Ø is prepared from the seeds.

Digestive disturbances and congestions are associated with this plant, flatulence and indigestion being commonly encountered. Stools are generally hard.

Ocimum Canum. N.O. Labiatae.
The Ø is prepared from the fresh leaves.

This remedy exerts its action mainly on the urinary system producing a turbid urine of a deep yellow colour. The urine itself is slimy and purulent with a musky sweet smell. Mainly used in urinary disturbances showing the typical symptoms.

Opium. Poppy. N.O. Papaveraceae.
The Ø is prepared from the powder after trituration.

Opium produces an insensibility of the nervous system with stupor and torpor. There is lack of vital reaction. All complaints are characterised by soporific states. Pupils are contracted and the eyes assume a staring look.

Ovarium.
This is also one of the ovarian hormones in potency. It covers a range of action similar to Folliculinum but the results have been shown to be less satisfactory than with the latter remedy.

Palladium. The Metal.
Potencies are prepared from triturations and subsequent dilution in alcohol.

This element produces its main action on the female genital system, especially the ovaries causing an inflammation with a tendency to pelvic peritonitis. The right ovary is more usually affected. Pelvic disorders arising as a result of ovaritis should also benefit.

Pancreas — Pancreatinum.
The Ø is prepared from pancreas extract after trituration.

It is used on various disorders of the pancreas either on its own or combined with selected remedies to suit the individual case. In pancreatitis it can be used along with the digestive enzyme Trypsin.

Pareira. Velvet Leaf. N.O. Menispermaceae.
The Ø is prepared from tincture of fresh root.

The active principle of this plant exerts its action mainly on the urinary system producing catarrhal inflammation of the bladder with a tendency to calculus formation. In the female there may be vaginal or uterine discharge. It is a useful remedy to consider in cases of vesical calculus where the animal is presented with acute strangury and distress.

Parotidinum.
This is the nosode of mumps and in veterinary practice it is a useful remedy in the treatment of cases of parotid gland swellings and associated structures. It may be used either on its own or combined with indicated remedies.

Petroleum. Rock Spirit.
The Ø is prepared from the oil.
This substance produces cutaneous eruptions and catarrhal mucous membranes. Eczematous eruptions develop around ears and eyelids and feet producing fissures which are slow to heal. The skin is usually dry. Complaints are usually worse in cold weather. A useful remedy for some forms of chronic skin conditions where symptoms agree.

Phosphoricum Acidum. Phosphoric Acid.
Potencies are prepared from a dilution of the acid in distilled water.
This acid produces a debilitating state in which flatulence and diarrhoea are common features.

Phosphorus. The Element.
The Ø is prepared from trituration of red phosphorus.
This important substance produces an inflammatory and degenerative effect on mucous membranes and causes bone destruction and necrosis of liver and other parenchymatous organs. It has a profound effect on eye structures especially the retina and iris. There is a marked haemorrhagic diathesis associated with this remedy, and small haemorrhages appear on skin and mucous membranes. Its uses in practice are wide and varied and it is one of the most important remedies in the pharmacopoeia.

Phytolacca Decandra. Poke Root. N.O. Phytolaccaceae.
The Ø is prepared from the whole fresh plant.

A state of restlessness and prostration is associated with this plant, together with glandular swellings. It is chiefly used in veterinary practice to combat swellings of the mammary glands in particular when the glands become hard and painful. Abscesses may develop together with mastitis of varying degree. In the male testicular swelling may occur. The remedy is of immense value in mastitis and other forms of mammary swellings.

Platina. The Metal Platinum.
The Ø is prepared from trituration of the metal with lactose.

This metal has a specific action on the female genital system, especially the ovaries where inflammation readily develops. Cystic ovaries develop frequently. This is a useful remedy to consider in certain breeds of cats e.g. Siamese, Birman and Burmese where the temperament appears to suit the psychological aspects of this remedy.

Plumbum Metallicum. The Metal Lead.
The Ø is prepared from trituration with sugar of milk.

A state of paralysis preceded by pain is produced by exposure to or ingestion with lead. It affects the central nervous system and also causes liver damage leading to jaundiced states. Blood pictures show anaemia. Paralyses of lower limbs develop and convulsions are common leading to coma. It should be remembered as a useful remedy to consider in degenerative renal states associated with liver involvement.

Podophyllum. May Apple. N.O. Ranuculaceae.
The Ø is prepared from the whole fresh plants.

The active principle of this plant exerts its action mainly on the duodenum and small intestine causing an enteritis. The liver and rectum are also affected. Distension of the abdomen occurs with a tendency to lie on the abdomen. Colicky pains develop with tenderness over the liver. A watery greenish diarrhoea may alternate with constipation. It is a useful remedy for gastro-intestinal disorders of young animals especially and for liver and portal congestion.

Psorinum. Scabies Vesicle.
The Ø is prepared from trituration of the dried vesicle.

This nosode produces a state of debility, especially after acute illness with skin symptoms predominating. All discharges are unpleasant. Chronic ophthalmia is occasionally seen along with otitis media and externa producing an offensive brownish discharge. Skin conditions are accompanied by severe itching. Animals needing this remedy prefer warmth.

Ptelea. Water Ash. N.O. Rutaceae.
The Ø is prepared from the bark or root.

This plant produces its main action on the stomach and liver. Hepatitis occurs with tenderness over liver and stomach areas. This is a good 'cleansing' remedy in that it will aid elimination of toxins and thereby help clear conditions such as eczema and asthmatic tendencies.

Pulsatilla. Anemone. N.O. Ranunculaceae.
The Ø is prepared from the entire plant when in flower.

Mucous membranes come within the sphere of action of this plant, thick muco-purulent discharges being produced. It has proved useful in the treatment of ovarian hypofunction and in retained placenta.

Pyrogenium. Artificial Sepsin.
The Ø is prepared from solutions of raw protein in distilled water.

This nosode has a specific relation to septic inflammations associated with offensive discharges. It is indicated in all septic conditions where the animal presents a clinical picture of raised temperature alternating with a weak thready pulse, or vice versa. It should be used in potencies of 200c and upwards.

Ranunculus Bulbosus. Buttercup. N.O. Ranunculaceae.
The Ø is prepared from the whole plant.

The action is mainly on muscular tissue and skin producing a hypersensitivity to touch. Skin lesions take the form of papular and vesicular eruptions which may cluster together into oval-shaped groups.

Rescue Remedy.
This is one of the many Bach Flower remedies and possibly the one most widely known and used. These remedies are not potentised like homoeopathic remedies but have been shown in practice to exert remarkable curative properties. Rescue Remedy is used to benefit the patient after exposure to any traumatic experience e.g. stress, shock and post-operative trauma. A very useful remedy to revive weak kittens after birth.

Rhododendron. Snow Rose. N.O. Ericaceae.
The Ø is prepared from the fresh leaves.
   This shrub is associated with muscular and joint stiffness. Orchitis is not uncommon with the testicles becoming hard and indurated.

Rhus Toxicodendron. Poison Oak. N.O. Anacardiaceae.
The Ø is prepared from the fresh leaves.
   The active principles of this tree affect skin and muscles together with mucous membranes and fibrous tissues producing tearing pains and blistery eruptions. Symptoms of stiffness are relieved by movement. Involvement of the skin leads to a reddish rash with vesicles and produces a cellulitis of neighbouring tissues. It could be a useful remedy in muscle and joint conditions which show a characteristic improvement on exercise.

Rumex Crispus. Yellow Dock. N.O. Polygonaceae.
The Ø is prepared from the fresh root.
   The active principle of this plant causes a diminution in the secretions from mucous membranes. Chronic gastritis occurs accompanied by an aversion to food and a watery diarrhoea. Mucous discharges take place from the trachea and nose. These tend to assume a frothy appearance. It is a useful remedy in some forms of respiratory affections.

Ruta Graveolens. Rue. N.O. Rutaceae.
The Ø is prepared from the whole fresh plant.
   Ruta produces its action on the periosteum and cartilages with a secondary effect on eyes and uterus. Deposits form around the carpal

47

joints, particularly. It has also a selective action on the lower bowel and rectum and could prove useful in mild forms of rectal prolapse. It has been known to facilitate labour by increasing the tone of uterine contractions.

Sabina. Savine. N.O. Coniferae.
The Ø is prepared from the oil dissolved in alcohol.

The uterus is the main seat of action producing a tendency to abortion. There is also an action of fibrous tissues and serous membranes. It is associated with haemorrhages of bright red blood which remains fluid. This remedy has its main use in uterine conditions including retained placenta. Persistent post-partum bleeding may also be arrested.

Sanguinaria. Blood Root. N.O. Papaveraceae.
The Ø is prepared from the fresh root.

An alkaloid — sanguinarine — contained in this plant has an affinity with the circulatory system leading to congestion and redness of skin. The female genital system is affected, inflammation of ovaries occurring. Small cutaneous haemorrhages arise in various sites. Stiffness of fore-legs, especially the left shoulder region may be seen.

Secale Cornutum. Ergot of Rye. N.O. Fungi.
The Ø is prepared from the fresh fungus.

Ergot produces marked contraction of smooth muscle causing a diminution of blood supply to various areas. This is particularly seen in peripheral blood vessels, especially of the feet. Stools are dark green alternating with dysentery. Bleeding of dark blood occurs from the uterus with putrid discharges. The skin becomes dry and shrivelled-looking with a tendency for gangrene to form. Because of its circulatory action and its effect on smooth muscle it is useful in some uterine conditions, e.g. post-partum bleeding of dark blood and in any condition with impairment of peripheral circulation.

Sepia Officinalis. Cuttlefish.
Potencies are prepared from trituration of the dried liquid from the ink bag.

Portal congestion and stasis are associated with this substance along with disturbances of function in the female genital system. Prolapse of uterus may occur or a tendency thereto. It will regulate the entire oestrus cycle and should always be given as a routine preliminary remedy in treatment. It has also an action on the skin and has given good results in the treatment of ringworm. Post-partum discharges of various sorts will usually respond. It is also capable of encouraging the natural maternal instinct in those animals which are indifferent or hostile to their offspring.

Silicea. Pure Flint.
Potencies are prepared from triturations dissolved in alcohol.
The main action of this substance is on bone where it is capable of causing caries and necrosis. It also causes abscesses and fistulae of connective tissue with secondary fibrous growths. There is a tendency for all wounds to suppurate. This is a widely used remedy indicated in many suppurative processes of a chronic nature.

Solidago Virga. Golden Rod. N.O. Compositae.
The Ø is prepared from the whole fresh plant.
This plant produces an inflammatory action on parenchymatous organs, particularly the kidney. The urine is scanty, reddish and accompanied by albumen deposits. Prostatic enlargement is frequently encountered. It is a useful remedy to consider in certain cases of renal insufficiency either with or without prostatic enlargement in the male animal.

Spigelia. Pink Root. N.O. Loganacea.
The Ø is prepared from the dried herb.
This plant has an affinity for the nervous system and also exerts an action on the cardiac region and the eye, producing ophthalmia and dilated pupils. A useful remedy for certain eye conditions especially if pain above the eyes can be elicited from the patient.

Spongia Tosta. Roasted Sponge.
Potencies are prepared from dilutions in alcohol.
This substance produces symptoms related to the respiratory and cardiac spheres. The lymphatic system is also affected. The thyroid

gland becomes enlarged. The general action on glands suggests its use in lymphadenitis. It is principally used as a heart remedy after respiratory infections.

Squilla Maritima. Sea Onion. N.O. Liliaceae.
The Ø is prepared from the dried bulb.

This substance acts especially on the mucous membranes of the respiratory tract. The digestive and renal systems are also affected. Nasal discharges develop accompanied by a dry cough which later becomes mucoid. There is urging to urinate, the urine being watery and profuse. It is a useful remedy for heart and kidney affections being especially valuable in dropsical conditions.

Staphisagria. Stavesacre. N.O. Ranunculaceae.
The Ø is prepared from the seeds.

The nervous system is mainly involved with this plant but there is also an action on the genito-urinary tract and the skin. A useful remedy in cystitis, but probably its most important indication is as a post-operative remedy where it acts on the mental level reducing psychological trauma and hastening the healing of wounds. It is also of benefit in the treatment of hormonal eczemas and alopecias.

Stramonium. Thorn Apple. N.O. Solanaceae.
The Ø is prepared from the whole fresh plant and fruit.

The active principle of this shrub produces its main action on the central nervous system, especially the cerebrum, producing a staggering gait with a tendency to fall forward on to the left side. Dilation of pupils occurs with a fixed staring look. A useful remedy to consider in brain disturbances where overall symptoms agree.

Streptococcus and Staphylococcus.
Streptococcus nosode is used in conditions associated with infections by this organism, e.g. erythematous rashes, tonsillitis and nephritis with associated pyelitis. It can be combined with other selected remedies. Staphylococcus aurens is the main remedy to consider in staphylococcal affections, e.g. abscesses and mastitis. These nosodes are used usually in 30c potency.

Strophanthus. Onage. N.O. Apocynaceae.
The Ø is prepared from the seeds dissolved in alcohol.

This shrub produces an increase in the contractile power of striped muscle. It acts especially on the heart increasing systole. The amount of urine passed is increased and albuminuria may be present. This is a useful heart remedy to help remove oedema. It is a safe and useful diuretic especially for the older animal.

Strychninum. Strychnine. Alkaloid Contained in Nux Vomica.
Potencies are prepared from solutions in distilled water.

This alkaloid stimulates the motor centres of the spinal cord and increases the depth of respirations. All reflexes are rendered more active and pupils become dilated. Rigidity of muscles occurs especially of the neck and back with jerking and twitching of limbs. Muscle tremors and tetanic convulsions set in rapidly.

Sulfonal. A derivative of Coal Tar.
The Ø is prepared from solution in alcohol or trituration with lactose.

This substance affects the central nervous system causing irregular movements, twitchings and incoordination of muscles which become stiff with a paralytic tendency. A useful remedy to consider in cases of cerebro-cortical affections showing the typical neuro-muscular symptoms.

Sulphur. The Element.
Potencies are prepared from trituration and subsequent dilution in alcohol.

This element has a wide range of action, but it is chiefly used in skin conditions such as mange and eczema and also as an inter-current remedy to aid the action of other remedies.

Symphytum. Comfrey. N.O. Boraginaceae.
The Ø is prepared from the fresh plant.

The root of this plant produces a substance which stimulates growth of epithelium on ulcerated surfaces and hastens union of bone in fractures. It should always be given as a routine remedy in fractures as an aid to healing. Together with other vulneraries like Arnica it is indicated in the treatment of injuries in general. It is also a prominent eye remedy.

Syzygium. Jumbul. N.O. Myrtaceae.
The Ø is prepared from trituration of seeds and subsequent dilution in alcohol.

This plant exerts an action on the pancreas and this defines its use in practice, especially in diabetes where it reduces the specific gravity of the urine and reduces thirst and controls output of urine.

Tabacum Tobacco.
This substance produces nausea and vomiting with intermittent pulse and weakness. In extreme cases there is a picture of muscular weakness and collapse.

Its main use in feline medicine would be in the treatment of sickness associated with movement, especially travel by sea.

Tarentula Hispanica. Spanish Spider.
The Ø is prepared from trituration of the whole insect.

Hysterical states are associated with this poison, and there is also a stimulatory action on the uro-genital system. A useful remedy to consider in cases of hysteria and epilepsy accompanied or preceded by excitement. Excessive libido (satyriasis) in the male may be helped.

Tellurium. The Metal.
The Ø is prepared from trituration with lactose.

This element exerts an influence on skin, eyes and ears. There is also an action on the sacral region. Cataracts and conjunctivitis develop. In the skin herpetic eruptions appear which assume an annular shape. This remedy is a useful one to consider in some forms of ear trouble where eruptions appear on the ear flap.

Terebinthinae. Oil of Turpentine.
Potencies are prepared from a solution in alcohol.

Haemorrhages are produced from various surfaces, urinary symptoms predominating. There is difficulty in urinating and blood commonly occurs in the urine. Bleeding may also take place in the uterus, especially after parturition. It is principally used in acute nephritis associated with haematuria and a sweet-smelling urine. This odour has been likened to that of violets. It also has a use in the treatment of gaseous bloat when low potencies will help.

Testosterone.
This is a male hormone secreted by the testicle and is used mainly in the treatment of miliary eczema and alopecia in the castrated male. It has been shown clinically to be less effective in this connection than the female hormones Folliculinum and Ovarium. It has also been used with varying success in the treatment of anal adenoma.

Thallium Acetas.
The metallic salt is triturated and dissolved in alcohol.
This metal exerts an action on the endocrine system and also on the skin and neuro-muscular system where it produces paralysis followed by muscular atrophy. The skin conditions frequently result in alopecia. It is used mainly in the treatment of trophic skin conditions e.g. chronic alopecia and myelitis.

Thlaspi Bursa Pastoralis. Shepherd's Purse. N.O. Cruciferae.
The Ø is prepared from the fresh plant.
This plant produces haemorrhages with a uric acid diathesis. It favours expulsion of blood clots from the uterus and is indicated after miscarriage. There is frequency of urination, the urine being heavy and turbid with a reddish sediment. Cystitis is commonly seen with blood-stained urine.

Thuja Occidentalis. Arbor Vitae. N.O. Coniferae.
The Ø is prepared from fresh twigs.
Thuja produces a condition which favours the formation of warty growths and tumours. It acts mainly on the skin and uro-genital system. Warts and herpetic eruptions develop, the neck and abdomen being the favourite sites. This remedy is of great importance in the treatment of skin conditions accompanied by the development of warty growths which bleed easily. Papillomatous warts are especially influenced and this action may be enhanced by the external application of the remedy in Ø form.

Thyroidium. Thyroid Gland.
Potencies are prepared from triturations and dilution in alcohol.

Anaemia, emaciation and muscular weakness are associated with excess of thyroid secretion. There is dilation of pupils with prominence. Heart rate is increased. This remedy may be of use in the treatment of alopecia and allied skin conditions.

Trinitrotoluene.
Potencies are prepared from a solution in distilled water.

This substance exerts a destructive influence on red blood cells causing haemolysis with consequent loss of haemoglobin. This produces anaemia and this is the principle of treatment by this remedy.

Tuberculinum Bovinum.
This nosode should be considered if a case of tuberculosis is encountered, but apart from this it is indicated in the treatment of osteomyelitis and some forms of peritonitis and pleurisy with effusions.

Uranium Nitricum. Uranium Nitrate.
The Ø is prepared from solution in distilled water.

Glycosuria and polyuria are the main objective symptoms associated with the provings of this salt. There is a marked action on the pancreas where it influences digestive function. Large amounts of urine are passed. This is a useful remedy in pancreatitis where it follows well after the remedy Iris versicolor.

Urtica Urens. Stinging Nettle. N.O. Urticaceae.
The Ø is prepared from the fresh plant.

The nettle causes agalactia with a tendency to the formation of calculi. There is a general uric acid diathesis with urticarial swellings being present on the skin. There is diminished secretion of urine. The mammary glands become enlarged with surrounding oedema. This is a very useful remedy in various renal and skin conditions. In the treatment of uric acid tendencies it acts by thickening the urine which contains increased deposits of urates.

Ustilago Maydis. Corn Smut. N.O. Fungi.
The Ø is prepared from trituration of the fungus with lactose.

This substance has an affinity for the genital organs of both sexes, particularly the female where the uterus is markedly affected. Alopecia of varying degrees develop accompanying a dry coat. Uterine bleeding occurs, the blood being bright red and partly clotted. Haemorrhages occur post-partum. In the male satyriasis occurs and this leads to one of its main uses in veterinary practice to control excessive sexual activity. The uterine action should not be overlooked.

Uva Ursi. Bearberry. N.O. Ericaceae.
The Ø is prepared from dried leaves and fruit.

The active principles are associated with disturbances of the urinary system. Cystitis commonly occurs and the urine may contain blood, pus and mucus. Kidney involvement is usually confined to the pelvis causing a purulent inflammation. This is one of the main remedies used in the treatment of cystitis and pyelonephritis.

Veratrum Album. White Hellebore. N.O. Liliaceae.
The Ø is prepared from root stocks.

A picture of collapse is presented by the action of this plant. Extremities become cold and signs of cyanosis appear. Purging occurs, the watery diarrhoea being accompanied by exhaustion. The body surface quickly becomes cold and the stools are greenish. Signs of abdominal pain precede the onset of diarrhoea.

Viburnum Opulus. Water Elder. Cranberry. N.O. Caprifoliaceae.
The Ø is prepared from the fresh bark.

Muscular cramps are associated with the action of this plant. The female genital system is markedly affected, chiefly the uterus producing a tendency to abortion in the first quarter of pregnancy, sterility being a common sequel. It is principally used in the treatment of animals with a history of repeated miscarriages.

Vipera. Common Viper.
Potencies are prepared from diluted venom.

This poison causes paresis of the hind limbs with a tendency to paralysis. Symptoms extend upwards. Skin and subcutaneous tissues become swollen after a bite with livid tongue and swollen lips developing. Disturbances of liver function produce a jaundice of visible mucous membranes. Inflammation of veins occurs with attendant oedema. Oedematous states arising from venous congestion provide conditions suitable for its use and it should be remembered as a possibly useful remedy in liver dysfunction.

Zincum Metallicum. Zinc. The Metal.
Potencies are prepared from trituration with subsequent dilution in alcohol.

This element produces a state of anaemia with a decrease in the number of red cells. There is a tendency to fall towards the left side with weakness and trembling of muscles. It is a useful remedy in suppressed feverish states accompanied by anaemia and may prove useful in brain conditions showing typical symptoms.

Nosodes and Oral Vaccines

Reference to nosodes and oral vaccines has already been made in the preface to this book, and it is only necessary to add that all disease products are rendered innocuous after the third centesimal potency which is equivalent to a strength or dilution of 1/1,000,000. They are used in the 30c potency.

Bacillinum.
This remedy is prepared from tuberculous material. It is extremely useful in the treatment of ringworm and similar skin diseases.

Carcinosin.
The Nosode of Carcinoma.

This little used remedy can be helpful in cases of glandular enlargements accompanied by feverish states.

E. Coli Nosode and Oral Vaccine.
Prepared from various strains of E. Coli. It has been found in practice that the strain which has given the most consistent results is the one which was prepared originally from a human source.

Folliculinum.
The nosode prepared from the corpus luteum is used chiefly in the treatment of various ovarian and allied conditions.

Oopherinum.
This is the actual ovarian hormone. Ovarian troubles come within its sphere of action, e.g. sterility dependent on ovarian dysfunction. It also has been used in some forms of skin disorder thought to be associated with hormone imbalance.

Psorinum. Scabies Vesicle.
This is a valuable skin remedy. Ringworm may respond as well as other conditions attended by dry coat and great itching.

Pyrogenium. Pyrogen.
This nosode is prepared from decaying animal protein. Despite its origin it is an extremely valuable remedy in the treatment of septicaemic or toxaemic states where vital reserves are low. One of the main indications for its use is illness attended by a high temperature alternating with a weak thready pulse, or alternatively a low temperature with a firm pulse. All discharges and septic states are extremely offensive. It could have a vital part to play in puerperal feverish conditions, and has been used in retained afterbirth after abortions.

Salmonella Nosode and Oral Vaccine.
Prepared from the common Salmonella organisms associated with this disease and used both prophylactically and therapeutically.

Streptococcus Nosode and Oral Vaccine.
Prepared from strains of haemolytic streptococci. It is used in various infections associated with these bacteria.

Sycotic Co. One of the Bowel Nosodes.
This is one of a group of nosodes prepared from the non-lactose fermenting bacilli found in the large intestine. Each one is related to certain homoeopathic remedies and used mainly in conjunction with

them. They are also used by themselves. Sycotic Co. has been used successfully in intestinal conditions producing catarrhal inflammation on mucous membranes.

Tuberculinum Aviare.
Avian sources provide the material for this nosode.

This nosode may prove useful in the treatment of some forms of pneumonia, along with indicated remedies. Chronic conditions are the most likely to benefit.

Diseases of the Alimentary System

1. STOMATITIS

Inflammation of the mouth. This may arise from various causes internal and external.

SYMPTOMS. The mouth appears red and swollen while ulcerative patches may be seen here and there. These leave a red raw surface which is painful on touch and subject to secondary infection when salivation may become purulent.

TREATMENT. If early cases are attended by a rise of temperature as is often the case then

1. ACONITUM. should be given as soon as possible. A single dose of 10m should be sufficient.

2. MERC SOL. One of the main keynotes of this remedy is profuse salivation. The mouth may appear dirty and there is usually nightly aggravation and symptoms. Suggested potency 6c, giving one dose three times daily for 5 days.

3. ACID NITRIC. Ulceration of the buccal mucous membrane is established when this remedy may be needed, especially when such ulceration occurs near the lips. Suggested potency 30c, giving one dose daily for 10 days.

4. BORAX. Indications for this remedy include the formation of vesicles as well as inflammatory changes. These vesicles tend to coalesce and then burst leaving a raw red surface. Salivation is excessive. A further indication for its use is a disinclination to move downwards e.g. coming off a chair or other high object. Suggested potency 6c, giving one dose three times daily for 7 days.

5. BELLADONNA. When this remedy is indicated the mouth is dry and presents a red shiny appearance. Concomitant signs include dilation of pupils and a full bounding pulse. The animal may feel hot. Suggested potency 1m, giving one dose hourly for 4 hours.

2. RANULA

This term denotes a cyst-like swelling beneath the tongue. It is usually caused by obstruction of a salivary duct.

SYMPTOMS. A globular swelling which may be one side or bilateral appears under the tongue.

TREATMENT. This is not easy by medicinal means but the following remedies may be helpful

1. APIS MEL. Indicated because of the oedematous nature of the condition. The patient is worse from heat and is usually thirstless. Suggested potency 6c, giving one dose three times daily for 7 days.

2. MERC SOL. If the condition is attended by excess salivation from other parts then this remedy may help. Suggested potency 6c, giving one dose three times daily for 5 days.

3. PAROTITIS. Inflammation of the Parotid Salivary Gland.

This condition may arise from exposure to cold and may also be a sequel to infectious disease such as F.V.R. (Feline Viral Rhino Tracheitis).

CLINICAL SIGNS. The condition is usually unilateral, and the gland becomes swollen, hard and painful.

TREATMENT. The following remedies should be considered

1. ACONITUM. Exposure to cold winds is an indication for the use of this remedy. Given early it may obviate the need for further treatment. Suggested potency 10m, giving one dose every 2 hours for 3 doses.

2. BELLADONNA. The gland becomes hot and swollen. There may be attendant signs of central nervous system involvement e.g. mild fits. Pupils will be dilated and the pulse full and bounding. General body heat is present. Suggested potency 1m, giving one dose hourly for four doses.

3. PULSATILLA. Indicated in those cases showing right sided involvement. The mouth is dry with a whitish coating to the tongue. Suggested potency 6c, giving one dose three times daily for 10 days.

4. BRYONIA. Hardness of the gland is a feature indicating this remedy, and like Aconite there is a history of exposure to cold. The patient is not averse to pressure on the gland. Mucous membranes (mouth) are dry. Suggested potency 30c, giving one dose twice daily for 7 days.

5. BARYTA CARB. If the condition affects very young or very old animals this remedy should be considered. There is a tendency for neighbouring tonsillar tissue to become involved. Suggested potency 6c, giving one dose three times daily for 7 days.

6. CALC FLUOR. Stony hardness developing in the gland calls for the remedy; associated lymph glands become involved. Suggested potency 30c, giving one dose twice weekly for 4 weeks.

7. PHYTOLACCA. This is a first class remedy for glandular involvement generally. The swelling extends to the throat which may become bluish-red causing difficulty in swallowing. More useful for acute states. Suggested potency 30c, giving one dose twice daily for 10 days.

8. RHUS TOX. The left parotid gland is normally affected if this remedy is indicated. Small vesicles may appear on the skin surrounding the gland and the throat becomes red and inflamed. Suggested potency 1m, giving one dose daily for 10 days.

9. PAROTIDINUM. The use of the nosode is indicated along with selected remedies. Suggested potency 30c, giving one dose daily for 5 days.

4. PHARYNGITIS. Inflammation of Throat.

Cold winds may again be implicated in the development of this condition. Occasionally change of food brings it on.

CLINICAL SIGNS. Difficulty in swallowing is usually the first thing that the owner notices. On examination there is tenderness to pressure over the throat area. Inflammation may extend to associated glands and to the ear.

TREATMENT

1. ACONITE. Indicated early on in the acute febrile stage. Suggested potency 10m, giving one dose hourly for 3 doses.

2. BELLADONNA. A most important throat remedy where general signs of dilated pupils, strong bounding pulse and pyrexia are present. The animal may be excitable. Suggested potency 1m, giving one dose hourly for 4 doses.

3. MERC CYAN. A membranous deposit may appear on the throat when this remedy is indicated. There are accompanying signs of generalised toxic involvement. Suggested potency 30c, giving one dose three times daily for 6 days.

4. AESCULUS. On examination the throat veins appear swollen and distended. Signs of hepatic (liver) disturbances may be present e.g. jaundice. Pressure over abdomen is resented. Suggested potency 30c, giving one dose three times daily for 6 days.

5. LACHESIS. A most important throat remedy when external examination reveals the area to be swollen and tender. Internal examination shows redness, swelling and possibly haemorrhagic involvement. Suggested potency 30c, giving one dose three times daily for 10 days.

6. BRYONIA. Like *ACONITE* exposure to cold winds is an indication for this remedy. Pressure over the area brings relief. Oral mucous membranes are dry. Suggested potency 30c, giving one dose three times daily for 7 days.

7. ALUMEN. Tonsillar tissue becomes hardened accompanying a general hardness of superficial lymph nodes elsewhere. Suggested potency 30c, giving one dose twice daily for 10 days.

8. RHUS TOX. Dark redness of throat is an indication for this remedy especially when the left side appears to be more involved than the right. Vesicles on tongue and gums accompany the condition. Suggested potency 1m, giving one daily for 10 days.

5. GINGIVITIS

This term indicates inflammation of the gums and apart from specific diseases (q.v.) this condition may appear in a non-specific form.

CLINICAL SIGNS. The gums appear red and swollen, the area adjacent to the teeth being more severely affected than others. Salivation is usually present: ulceration may or may not be a feature.

TREATMENT

1. MERC SOL. Simple inflammation showing excessive saliva may be helped by this remedy. There is a general dirty look to the mouth and a nightly exacerbation of symptoms occurs. Suggested potency 6c, giving one dose three times daily for 10 days.

2. MERC IOD RUB. The double valency of mercury yields an iodide which has a beneficial effect on inflammation affecting the left side of the mouth. Suggested potency 30c, giving one dose three times daily for 7 days.

3. MERC IOD FLAV. The yellow iodide of mercury acts in a similar fashion but has a predilection for the right side. Suggested potency 30c, giving one dose three times daily for 7 days.

4. BORAX. Ulceration is present when this remedy is indicated. Salivation is excessive and patients exhibit a disinclination to jump down from chairs etc. or go downstairs. Suggested potency 6c, giving one dose twice daily for 14 days.

5. MERC CORR. Somewhat similar in its indications to Merc Sol but symptoms are much more severe. There may be an accompanying nightly mucous slimy stool. Suggested potency 30c, giving one dose twice daily for 7 days.

6. GLOSSITIS. Inflammation of tongue.

Simple inflammation is occasionally seen in cats when presenting signs include a red shiny appearance, the animal being unwilling to lap or eat because of tenderness of the epithelium. Remedies such as *BELLADONNA* 1m potency three times a day for 4 days and *RHUS*

TOX 1m used in the same way may help. Specific disease/ulcerative glossitis is discussed in the chapter on diseases due to infective agents.

7. GASTRITIS. Inflammation of stomach.

In cats trouble of this nature is invariably due to impaction by fur balls or furry material which the animal has been unable to expel in the normal way. Other agents may also contribute.

SYMPTOMS. The cat exhibits signs of uneasiness and inappetance and attempts may be made to vomit. The condition is relatively mild in cats and remedies such as *NUX VOM* 6c one dose three times daily for 3 days should help. This is a reliable remedy for simple indigestion and should stimulate the appetite. Gastritis due to ingestion of foreign material may occur occasionally but less likely in this species than in the dog. If this leads to vomiting with pain the remedy *PHOSPHORUS* should be considered, giving a dose of 30c potency every 2 hours for 4 doses.

8. ENTERITIS AND DIARRHOEA

Apart from specific enteritis (q.v.) a non-specific form may affect young kittens yielding loose stools of a light colour and foul odour. These young animals showing such a syndrome should benefit from one or other of the following remedies.

1. GAERTNER. This bowel nosode is indicated generally in enteric conditions of young animals as a preliminary remedy which complements other related ones. Suggested potency 30c, giving one dose daily for 5 days.

2. E. COLI. This nosode may also be needed and can be combined with the previous one giving it in the same way. It is a good practice when faced with this condition in kittens to have a specific nosode made from faecal material.

2. BARYTA CARB. This is a remedy which suits very young animals and should be kept in mind as a complementary remedy to be given if response to others is slow. Suggested potency 6c, giving one dose three times daily for 7 days.

4. CHINA. Always indicated when loss of body fluid occurs. Again may be used in conjunction with other remedies. Suggested potency 6c, giving a dose 4 – 5 times daily for 2 days.

5. VER ALB. If the condition is severe leading to collapse this remedy may have to be considered. Stools are described as like rice-water. suggested potency 30c, giving one dose three times daily for 5 days.

6. PODOPHYLLUM. A useful remedy in long-standing cases which have not shown response to other remedies. Particularly useful in young animals showing a morning aggravation. Suggested potency 1m, giving one dose daily for 6 days.

9. CONSTIPATION

This may be due to many factors and should be dealt with by strict attention to diet ensuring that plenty of bulk is available in the food together with a proper fluid intake. The condition may be associated with systemic illnesses when constitutional remedies may be needed.

Remedies to consider in alleviating the condition are:

1. NUX VOM. Digestive disturbances generally. Vomiting may take place accompanying flatulence and tenderness over liver region. Suggested potency 6c, giving one dose three times daily for 7 days.

2. ALUMEN. Frequent vomiting accompanies involvement of the lymphatic glands which become typically hard. Suggested potency 30c, giving one dose daily for 7 days.

3. NAT MUR. A most useful constitutional remedy for cats generally. Vesicles may appear in the mouth and excessive drinking may accompany a general weakness. Suggested potency 6c – 9c – 200c.

4. BRYONIA. Stools are hard and appear as having a burnt look. The patient prefers rest and is disinclined to move. Mucous membranes are dry. Suggested potency 6c, giving one dose three times daily for 10 days.

5. *LYCOPODIUM.* When the condition is thought to accompany liver involvement. Symptoms generally worse about afternoon. May accompany respiratory difficulties. Suggested potency 12c, giving one dose twice daily for 14 days.

10. COLITIS

Inflammation of the large bowel is uncommon apart from the specific cases of feline enteritis. Symptoms may show as chronic diarrhoea of varying colour and consistency, and may be dependant on an ulcerative state of the epithelium of the gut. The following remedies all have a place in treatment depending on particular symptoms presented, and the character of the patient.

1. *IRIS VERS.* There may be accompanying swelling of throat region. Stools are generally yellowish or creamy. Suggested potency 30c, giving one dose daily for 10 days.

2. *MERC CORR.* Severe straining accompanies stools which are typically mucous and blood-stained. The condition is worse from sunset to sunrise. Suggested potency 30c, giving one dose twice daily for 7 days.

3. *ACID NIT.* If ulceration is suspected, especially of lower colon and/ or rectal involvement is prominent this remedy may help. Suggested potency 200c, giving one dose three times weekly for 4 weeks.

4. *URAN NIT.* If vomiting occurs after drinking this may be needed. Abdominal discomfort is accompanied by flatulence. Suggested potency 30c, giving one dose daily for 14 days.

5. *CROTON TIG.* Severe purgation is accompanied by skin symptoms such as excessive itching: skin feels hot. Stools very watery. Suggested potency 200c, giving one dose three times weekly for 3 weeks.

6. *IPECAC.* Associated with frequent vomiting: there may also be respiratory symptoms such as reflex vomiting associated with abdominal discomfort. Stools may contain blood. Suggested potency 6c, giving one dose three times daily for 10 days.

7. *DULCAMARA*. If the condition is associated with a history of patient having been exposed to wet conditions: also a seasonal association (Autumn). Suggested potency 200, giving one dose daily for 10 days.

8. *COLOCYNTH*. Severe signs of colic are associated. Patient cries out and arches back. May roll on ground and strain. Pain usually severe. Suggested potency 1m, giving one dose hourly for 4 doses.

9. *ARSEN ALB*. Foul-smelling stools described as cadaverous. Frequent drinking. Worse towards midnight. Animal restless. Dry coat: vomiting. Seeks heat. Suggested potency 1m, giving one dose twice daily for 4 days.

11. PROCTITIS

Inflammation of the rectal area may follow as a result of acute colitis or feline enteritis when profusion of rectal mucous membrane may occur.

Remedies such as *NUX VOM* 30c daily for 7 days and *RUTA* three times daily for 10 days may help as both have a part to play in this particular type of inflammation.

12. THE LIVER

(a) **Hepatitis** Inflammation of liver parenchyma may arise from time to time in cats when the patient is usually presented with a history of bilious vomiting and producing grey or clay-coloured stools. Jaundice (which is merely a symptom) may or may not be present and if so then stools may show as golden-yellow. A toxic form may arise from the ingestion accidentally of chemicals or from overdosing with certain chemical drugs.

TREATMENT. Depending on presenting signs the following remedies are indicated

1. *PHOSPHORUS*. A most useful remedy. Stools clay-coloured. Vomiting of water etc. May be accompanied by signs of bleeding gums. Suggested potency 30c, giving one dose twice daily for 6 days.

2. CHELIDONIUM. Jaundice usually accompanies. Mucous membranes yellow. Stools golden-yellow. Suggested potency 30c, giving one dose twice daily for 7 days.

3. LYCOPODIUM. More chronic cases showing indigestion and flatulence. Old subjects generally, aggravation of symptoms in late afternoon. Suggested potency 12c, giving one dose twice daily for 7 days: 1m giving one dose weekly for 4 weeks.

4. BERBERIS. If there is an accompanying loin weakness. Smell in urine. Biley colic. Suggested potency 30c, giving one dose daily for 10 days.

5. CHIONANTHUS. Liver usually palpable. Jaundice: putty-like stools. Suggested potency 6c, giving one dose three times daily for 10 days.

(b) Cirrhosis. The term implies chronic thickening of the liver parenchyma leading to a hardening which can be felt on external examination. It is of fairly frequent occurrence in the cat. Symptoms include also constipation, vomiting and the presence in the abdominal cavity of large amounts of fluid in severe cases. This arises from disturbances of the portal circulation.

TREATMENT

1. CARDUUS MAR. This is one of the main remedies to consider as it has a proven record in alleviating the condition. Constitutionally the animal will be much more alert and take more interest in its surroundings and in food. Suggested potency 30c, giving one dose twice daily for 14 days.

2. PHOSPHORUS. If food and water are rejected shortly after ingestion this remedy should be considered. It has a profound action on the liver function. Suggested potency 200c, giving one dose twice weekly for 4 weeks.

3. LYCOPODIUM. Another valuable liver remedy for the older animal and one which shows a worsening of symptoms in late afternoon and early evening. Stools are usually dry and shiny. Suggested potency 200c, giving one dose three times weekly for 3 weeks.

4. BERBERIS. This remedy may help in providing stimulation of the portal circulation leading to reduction of abdominal fluid. Its action on the kidneys will further help in this connection. Suggested potency 30c, giving one dose daily for 10 days.

5. PTELEA. A less well known remedy which has a beneficial action on the liver by acting as what is known as a drainage remedy, i.e. it helps cleanse the system in those cases where the liver (the main 'cleansing' organ) is not functioning normally. Suggested potency 30c, giving one dose twice daily for 14 days.

13. THE SPLEEN

Pathological conditions of the spleen in cats are invariably associated with the FeLV virus (q.v.). One particular remedy which aids splenic function is *CEANOTHUS* and a course of this remedy in 30c potency daily for 14 days may help if pathological involvement of this organ is suspected or diagnosed.

14. THE PANCREAS, PANCREATITIS ACUTE AND CHRONIC

The two functions of the pancreas viz. digestive and hormonal must be differentiated and treated as separate entities.

(a) Digestive function. This concerns the role of the amino-acid trypsin and its function in the digestion of protein.

CLINICAL SIGNS. A cat presented with the particular deficiency may show one or all of the following symptoms, viz. persistent diarrhoea the faeces being yellowish due to fat content, ravenous appetite and occasionally large stools containing undigested food. Loss of condition is apparent in long-standing cases.

TREATMENT. ACUTE FORM
1. IRIS VERS. This is a most important pancreatic remedy. Stools are watery and light coloured, or sometimes greenish. Abdominal pain is

severe. Suggested potency 6c, giving one dose three times daily for 5 days, followed by 30c potency, giving one dose three times weekly for 4 weeks.

2. ATROPINUM. The alkaloid of belladonna has a selective action on the pancreas and may be indicated in those cases associated with a dry mouth and inability to swallow properly. Vomiting relieves symptoms and the umbilical area is extremely sensitive to touch. Suggested potency 6c, giving one dose three times daily for 7 days.

3. CHIONANTHUS. This is a good general pancreatic remedy indicated when there are accompanying liver derangements showing clay-coloured stools and tenderness over the hepatic region. Abdominal pain is severe. Suggested potency 30c, giving one dose daily for 10 days.

4. IODUM. Stools are consistently frothy and fatty when this remedy is indicated. Suitable for the lean animal which shows a voracious appetite and dry coat. Suggested potency 30c, giving one dose daily for 2 weeks.

5. GAERTNER. This bowel nosode will aid the action of other selected remedies. Especially useful in the young animal. Suggested potency 30c, giving one dose daily for 5 days.

6. PANCREAS. The pancreas nosode will be found to be of use along with selected remedies. Suggested potency 30c, giving one dose daily for 7 days.

CHRONIC FORM. This may be associated with fibrous induration of pancreatic tissue and sometimes occurs as a sequal to the acute form.

CLINICAL SIGNS. The appetite is usually maintained and in many instances becomes excessive. Despite this, however, the animal suffers a progressive loss of weight. Thirst is also increased. A distinctive sign is the production of massive faecal bulk which is greyish in colour and fatty in consistency. Abdominal pain may be present but is not a constant sign.

TREATMENT. The following remedies have all proved useful according to individual symptoms

1. IODUM. This remedy is associated with voracious appetite and an inability to gain weight. It is well adapted to lean animals with dry harsh coats. Stools are frothy and contain fat globules. Lymphatic glands are often hard and smaller than usual. Suggested potency 30c, giving one dose daily for 14 days.

2. SILICEA. If it is suspected that fibrous tissue induration is present this remedy should prove useful. It has a deserved reputation in reducing scar or fibrous tissue. Suggested potency 200, giving one dose twice weekly for 6 weeks.

3. BARYTA CARB. This is a useful remedy for the older animal. Tonsillar tissue is frequently enlarged causing difficulty in swallowing and there may be intermittent vomiting. 6c twice daily for 7 days.

4. APOCYNUM CANNABINUM. Dropsical conditions such as ascites are usually present when this remedy is indicated. Thirst is markedly increased and persistent vomiting may be noticed. Suggested potency 30c, giving one dose daily for 14 days.

5. PHOSPHORUS. There is usually an accompanying hepatitis when phosphorus is indicated. Stools are clay-coloured and sago-like. Food and water are vomited shortly after ingestion. Small haemorrhages may appear on the mucous membranes of the mouth. Suggested potency 200c, giving one dose three times weekly for 4 weeks.

(b) Hormonal function - Diabetes. Sometimes affects older cats particularly neutered males. The portion of the pancreas which secretes insulin may become deficient in this respect leading to a shortage of this hormone which is essential to the metabolism of sugar and carbohydrates.

SYMPTOMS. Cats may be presented with a history of increased drinking and passing of urine. Wasting is a common sequal in established cases and occasionally opacity of lens (cataract) may develop but more rarely than in the dog.

TREATMENT. In severe cases the insulin deficiency must be overcome by the appropriate administration of this hormone. Milder cases may respond to a combination of diet and remedies which help regulate the function of the pancreas generally. Among these are

1. SYZYGIUM. This remedy has a pancreatic function and should be given in potency e.g. 1x – 3x three times daily for 21 days. This may have to be repeated after a period of 2 weeks or so and the response monitored thereafter.

2. URAN NIT. General dropsy and emaciation accompany the need for this remedy. Increased urination is present and mucous membranes become dry. Abdominal bloating is prominent. Suggested potency 30c, giving one dose three times weekly for 6 weeks.

3. IRIS VERS. Also indicated when there are loose light-coloured stools. Acts well on pancreas. Suggested potency 30c, giving one dose daily for 14 days.

Diseases of the Respiratory System

Many diseases of this system are part of the overall picture of specific diseases e.g. Feline Viral Rhonotracheitis and Calici Virus infection and reference should be made to these under the appropriate heading. The following non-specific conditions are the ones most likely to be encountered:

1. RHINITIS

This is the name given to the inflammation of the nasal mucous membrane and occurs only rarely as a separate entity. It is more often an accompaniment of specific diseases.

ETIOLOGY. The inflammatory process is usually started by some irritant factor but secondary infection soon sets in which changes the character of the discharge. Staphylococcal or Streptococci are usually implicated in these cases.

CLINICAL SIGNS. Nasal discharge is a constant sign. This starts as serous and thin becoming in stages mucous and finally muco-purulent. Streaks of blood may be present. The dischange may be acrid in which excoriation of the nostrils will be seen, and when persistent muco-purulent discharges are present they impede breathing because of obstruction of nostrils.

TREATMENT. Various remedies are available and these include the following
1. ARSENICUM ALBUM. This is a useful remedy in the early stages when the discharge is thin and excoriating. There may be an accompanying watery discharge from the eyes and also thirst for small quantities of water. The coat may be dry and harsh while symptoms tend to be exacerbated towards midnight. Suggested potency 30c, giving one dose daily for 10 days.

73

2. PULSATILLA. Mild-tempered animals showing changeable moods may respond to this remedy. Discharges are thick and bland. There may be an ulceration of the nostrils and small streaks of blood may show. Suggested potency 30c, giving one dose daily for 7 days.

3. MERC SOL. The discharge associated with this remedy assumes a greenish tinge and may contain blood. The nasal bones are frequently swollen. Symptoms are worse in the period from sunset to sunrise. Suggested potency 6c, giving one dose three times daily for 7 days.

4. ALLIUM CEPA. Discharges are thin and watery accompanied by sneezing and lachrymation. Suggested potency 6c, giving one dose three times daily for 3 days.

5. KALI IODATUM. This is a useful remedy for those cases where the discharge becomes impacted and there is an attempt to sneeze which is usually ineffectual. Watering of eyes is a prominent sign. Suggested potency 6c, giving one dose three times daily for 5 days.

6. KALI BICHROMICUM. Discharges assume a bright yellow colour and develop into small plugs which have a tough stringy appearance. Streaks of blood are often present. Suggested potency 30c, giving one dose daily for 10 days.

7. ACIDUM FLORICUM. If the nasal septum is suspected as a cause e.g. ulceration this remedy may be indicated. Suggested potency 12c, giving one dose twice daily for 14 days.

2. EPISTAXIS

Nose bleeding is rarely seen as an independent condition, most cases being due to mechanical injury. Occasionally it follows severe inflammatory lesions affecting the turbinate bones or upper nasal mucous membrances. The presence of tumours in the nasal cavity may also give rise to bleeding. Other cases again are a sequal to specific disease q.v.

TREATMENT. The following remedies have all proved effective according to the nature of the bleeding and overall symptoms presented:

1. ACONITUM. Indicated in spontaneous haemorrhage of bright red blood which could be the result of exposure to severe cold or shock. Suggested potency 10m, giving one dose every hour for 3 doses.

2. FICUS RELIGIOSA. This remedy covers haemorrhages generally and could be associated with haemorrhages elsewhere. Suggested potency 6c, giving one dose three times a day for 3 days.

3. PHOSPHORUS. Associated with small capillary bleeding from nasal mucous membranes rather than with a large flow of blood. Suggested potency 30c, giving one dose three times daily for 2 days.

4. CROTALUS HORR. The snake venoms as a group are associated with haemorrhages and bleeding may take place from other orifices. The blood has a tendency to remain fluid. Suggested potency 200, giving one dose daily for 5 days.

5. VIPERA. This remedy has an action somewhat similar to the previous remedy but has a greater tendency to vertigo. Suggested potency 1m, giving one dose daily for 7 days.

6. MELILOTUS. The blood is bright red and may accompany a feverish state. Blood coagulates in the nostrils in many cases. Suggested potency 30c, giving one dose daily for 7 days.

7. IPECACUANHA. This remedy also is associated with bright red blood. There are usually accompanying digestive upsets such as persistent vomiting when this remedy is indicated. Suggested potency 30c, giving one dose twice daily for 5 days.

8. FERRUM PHOSPH. Indicated more in kittens and frequently accompanied by difficult swallowing and possibly a feverish state. Suggested potency 6c, giving one dose three times daily for 3 days.

3. SINUSITIS

The sinuses occasionally become the seat of infection or inflammation resulting in a collection of purulent material within the sinus. The condition leads to nasal discharges of an offensive nature which can be difficult to treat, but the following remedies may prove useful:

1. HEPAR SULPH. Indicated when there is pain elicited by pressure over the sinus area. Low potencies will promote expulsion of pus (e.g.

6c) while higher potencies (e.g. 200) will promote granulation of the sinus linings. Three times daily for low potencies and three times per week for 4 weeks for higher ones.

2. *SILICEA*. Indicated in chronic states where there is less sensitivity. Suggested potency 200c, giving one dose three times weekly for 4 weeks.

3. *HIPPOZAENINUM*. This nosode has proved of value in chronic stages showing a honey-coloured sticky discharge. Suggested potency 3c, giving one dose daily for 10 days.

4. *LEMNA MINOR*. Discharges are extremely offensive and dirty and are accompanied by frequent sneezing. Suggested potency 6c, giving one dose three times daily for 5 days.

4. TONSILLITIS

Inflammation of tonsillar tissue is of fairly common occurence and may be acute or chronic.

(a) Acute form. This is associated with infection, mainly streptococcal although specific viruses are also responsible.

CLINICAL SIGNS. The affected tissue becomes swollen and reddened due to increased blood supply and may show greyish spots of necrosis and frothy exudate. Sometimes these spots coalesce to form a membrane which covers the tonsils. Appetite is variable but any attempt at swallowing is attended with discomfort. Saliva may be clean or mucoid. Retching is a frequent accompaniment with vomiting of excess mucus. A rise of temperature is usual in the early stages especially in kittens.

TREATMENT. The following remedies should be considered:

1. *ACONITUM*. Should be given as early as possible when it will probably prevent complications developing. Suggested potency 10m, giving three doses one hour apart.

2. *MERC CYAN*. The mercury remedies generally have a beneficial effect on mouth and throat conditions and this one in particular has a

proven value in thoat infections. Suggested potency 30c, giving one dose twice daily for 3 days.

3. PHYTOLACCA. Indicated when there is enlargement of tonsillar tissue and the throat has a dark red colour. Membranous deposits may be present along with a yellowish mucus. Suggested potency 30c, giving one dose twice daily for 7 days.

4. BELLADONNA. A most useful remedy appearing to act better when following *ACONITUM.* Animals show dilated pupils and have a strong bounding pulse. Temperature is usually raised. Suggested potency 6c, giving one dose three times daily for 3 days.

5. RHUS TOX. The tonsillar area shows a large amount of mucus and assumes a dark red colour. Externally the throat may be swollen. There may be accompanying eye symptoms such as lachrymation and swollen eyelids. Suggested potency 1m, giving one dose daily for 14 days.

6. LACHESIS. This snake venom remedy is frequently indicated in throat conditions. The tonsillar tissue appears dark blush-red or purple and considerable swelling is present. The condition appears to be aggravated after sleep. Suggested potency 12c, giving one dose three times daily for 5 days.

(b) Chronic Form. This can be the sequel to one or other of the virus diseases q.v. from which the animal has shown a recovery from the acute phase. Tonsils become enlarged while exacerbations are common, mild forms alternating with more severe manifestations.

The following remedies may prove useful:

1. SILICEA. This remedy will promote absorption of any fibrous or scar tissue and will also control any tendency to suppuration. Suggested potency 200c, giving one dose twice weekly for 6 weeks.

2. BARYTA CARB. Both very young and old subjects will benefit from this remedy. There is a marked tendency to suppuration of tonsillar tissue. Suggested potency 6c, giving one dose three times daily for 5 days.

3. CALCAREA IOD. This remedy has proved extremely useful in chronic tonsillitis where the tonsils remain enlarged and become pitted with superficial ulcers. The patient is likely to be lean with a dry coat. Suggested potency 30c, giving one dose daily for 10 days.

4. HEPAR SULPH. Tonsils which show purulent infection from time to time will be helped by this remedy. The throat becomes painful and sensitive to external pressure. Suggested potency 30c, giving one dose daily for 10 days.

5. KALI BICH. Swollen tonsils becoming ulcerated and yielding a yellow stringy pus are indications for this remedy. The tissue assumes a reddish-coppery tinge. Suggested potency 200c, giving one dose twice weekly for 6 weeks.

6. STREPTOCOCCUS. This nosode can profitably be combined with any of the foregoing remedies. A dose of 30c daily for 5 days should suffice.

5. LARYNGITIS

This condition may arise because of bacterial or viral invasion or it may arise in a sporadic fashion from other causes. There are varying degrees of severity encountered some proving fatal because of occlusion of air passages.

CLINICAL SIGNS. The owner's attention is first alerted by the cat making gulping noises as though some obstruction were present. There is a loss of voice or change in its character. Pressure over the laryngeal area is resented. Severe cases show extreme difficulty in breathing, the mouth being kept open.

TREATMENT. The cat should be kept in a quiet place and one or other of the following remedies considered:

1. ACONITUM. If given early in the condition the symptoms will be abated and the process halted. Suggested potency 10m, giving one dose every hour for 3 doses.

2. BELLADONNA. Indicated for the cat which shows excitability, full bounding pulse and dilated pupils. Suggested potency 12c, giving one dose every hour for 4 doses.

3. APIS MEL. If the inflammatory process is attended with much oedema this remedy should help. The animal is thirstless and there is an aversion to warmth. Suggested potency 30c, giving one dose three times daily for 3 days.

4. SPONGIA. Indicated in laryngeal conditions where a harsh croupous cough is prominent. There is an absence of mucus. Respiration is accompanied by a whistling sound. Suggested potency 6c, giving one dose three times daily for 7 days.

5. DROSERA. Spasmodic cough indicates this remedy. Hoarseness is very pronounced as also is tenacious mucus. The cough produces retching and vomiting and greatly impedes proper breathing. Suggested potency 9c, giving one dose three times per day for 7 days.

4. CAUSTICUM. Indicated in those cases where the voice becomes lost due to a temporary paralysis of the laryngeal nerves. The cough may excite urination. Mucus gathers in the throat with great difficulty in expelling. Suggested potency 30c, giving one dose twice daily for 10 days.

7. RHUS TOX. Indicated when the larynx is deep red and the cough is attended by greenish mucus of a putrid nature. Occasionally blood is present in the expectoration. A generalised stiffness of movement may be present. Suggested potency 1m, giving one dose daily for 12 days.

A chronic form of this condition may arise as a result of neglected cases or those subjected to maltreatment. It is characterised by hypertrophy of laryngeal tissue often with a membranous deposit covering the larynx. Narrowing of the laryngeal opening may develop. In addition to the foregoing remedies the following additional ones should be considered.

1. SILICEA. This remedy helps promote healing of fibrous or scar tissue and should guard against infection developing. Suggested potency 200, giving one dose twice weekly for 6 weeks.

2. CALC FLUOR. This is a good general tissue remedy and should aid healing. Suggested potency 30c, giving one dose three times per week for 4 weeks.

3. BARYTA MUR. A varicose condition of the throat veins is usually present when this remedy is indicated. There is a tendency to suppuration. Suggested potency 6c, giving one dose three times daily for 10 days.

6. BRONCHITIS

There is a seasonal association in connection with this trouble, cases being seen more frequently in the early and later parts of the year.

CLINICAL SIGNS. The chief symptom or sign is coughing which can vary in severity.

Rattling sounds may sometimes be heard. Appetite is usually maintained and there is little or no febrile involvement.

TREATMENT

1. BRYONIA. This remedy is indicated when the animal is better resting. Pressure over the affected area gives relief. Suggested potency 6c, giving one dose three times per day for 7 days.

2. KALI BICH. This is a useful remedy where excess mucus of a stringy yellow nature is expectorated. There may be an accompanying nasal discharge. Suggested potency 200c, giving one dose three times per week for 4 weeks.

3. ANTIMONIUM TART. When this remedy is indicated rattling of mucus is a prominent symptom, the discharge being frothy and mucoid. Suggested potency 30c, giving one dose twice daily for 10 days.

4. APIS MEL. When excess fluid is suspected leading to expectoration of fluid mucus, this remedy may help. Suggested potency 6c, giving one dose three times daily for 10 days.

5. SPONGIA. This is a useful remedy in the older animal when there are accompanying symptoms of heart involvement. Suggested potency 6c, giving one dose three times daily for 10 days.

6. RUMEX. This is an alternative remedy to the last named remedy. Mucus is excessive and the cough is relieved in the evening or during the night. Suggested potency 6c, giving one dose three times daily for 10 days.

7. SCILLA. Symptoms of gastric involvement e.g. vomiting and reflex coughing indicate this remedy. Suggested potency 6c, giving one dose three times daily for 7 days.

8. COCCUS CACTI. Coughing is present in a spasmodic nature in the earlier stages of the condition and is worse at night. Suggested potency 6c, giving one dose three times daily for 7 days.

7. BRONCHIECTASIS

This is the term used to describe the bronchial tree when it becomes abnormally dilated due to a loss of tone or elasticity in its fibres. This allows fluid to develop in pockets which eventually become receptacles for purulent material.

It is frequently a sequel to some other pulmonary disease, but it can also arise as a result of foreign bodies being aspirated into the lining. The primary disease is bacterial or viral in origin.

CLINICAL SIGNS. Continual coughing is the usual premonitory sign and while this is dry and unproductive in the early stages it soon becomes moist and the patient coughs up large quantities of muco-purulent material. A general loss of condition ensues.

TREATMENT

1. BRYONIA. This remedy may help in the early dry and unproductive stage. the animal resents movement and pressure over the chest brings relief. Suggested potency 6c, giving one dose three times daily for 3 days.

2. ANT TART. A useful remedy in the early stages after the exudate becomes frothy and rattling signs are heard. Suggested potency 30c, giving one dose twice daily for 5 days.

3. HEPAR SULPH. In the early purulent stage this remedy should limit the risk of secondary bacterial involvement. Suggested potency 30c, giving one dose twice daily for 7 days.

4. KALI BICH. Indicated when the cough is accompanied by tough mucus of a'yellow stringy nature. Suggested potency 200c, giving one dose three times per week for 3 weeks.

5. KREOSOTUM. A useful remedy in long-standing cases when gangrenous changes are threatened. The expectoration is extremely putrid and may be tinged with blood. Suggested potency 200c, giving one dose three times per week for 4 weeks.

6. MERC SOL. This remedy may be needed when any material coughed up is of a greenish rather than a yellow colour. Suggested potency 6c, giving one dose three times daily for 10 days.

Diseases of Lungs and Pleura

1. PULMONARY OEDEMA

An abmormal accumulation of fluid in the lung is usually a sequel to chronic heart disease, especially mitral valve insufficiency when the circulatory weakness leads to a transudation of blood plasma from the pulmonary veins into the lung tissue.

CLINICAL SIGNS. There is great difficulty in breathing and a moist cough is fairly constant. The cat may be seen in sternal recumbency with its head extended in order to obtain ease of breathing.

TREATMENT

1. APIS MEL. This remedy is always indicated when oedema is present. It should aid resorption and thereby give some relief. Suggested potency 6x, giving one dose 3 – 4 times daily for 10 days.

2. STROPHANTHUS. This heart remedy is indicated as it stimulates the heart action and will hasten output of urine and thereby help to reduce the fluid. Suggested potency 3x, giving one dose twice daily for 30 days.

3. ADONIS VER 3x. This is one of the best heart remedies where valvular insufficiency is present. Suggested potency 3x, giving one dose three times daily for 30 days.

4. CRATAEGUS. This heart remedy exerts its action on the muscle of the heart thereby increasing the force of the beat and leading to greater output of blood. In this way circulation as a whole is stimulated. Suggested potency 3x, giving one dose three times daily for 30 days.

5. CARBO VEG. This is a useful remedy which gives relief by helping the patient's oxygen supply and thereby aiding breathing. Suggested potency 200c, giving one dose daily for 7 days as necessary. It should be given preferably in the evening.

6. ABROTANUM. This remedy has a reputation for aiding conditions which give rise to exudations in general. It is therefore worth considering as a standby remedy if others do not appear to help. Suggested potency 6x, giving one dose three times daily for 14 days.

2. EMPHYSEMA

When the alveoli of the lungs lose their elasticity, becoming distended and unable to return to normal size, a state of emphysema is said to exist. In severe cases the alveolar wall may rupture permitting the escape of air into the surrounding tissues.

It is invariably a sequel to some chronic respiratory disorder such as bronchitis or cronchiectasis.

CLINICAL SIGNS. There is obvious difficulty in expelling air, and respiration may be associated with forced movements of the abdominal muscles in order to assist the process. There is general difficulty in breathing.

TREATMENT

1. LOBELIA INF. This remedy has proved useful in the treatment of functional emphysema where the changes in the alveolar walls have not proceeded too far or have become chronic. Suggested potency 30c, giving one dose twice daily for 14 days.

2. ANT ARSEN. This is a useful remedy when examination reveals that the left lung is affected more than the right. Suggested potency 30c, giving one dose twice daily for 10 days.

3. CARBO VEG. This remedy helps provide oxygen by its ability to help in cases of air hunger. It will give relief particularly at night. Suggested potency 200c, giving one dose each evening as necessary.

The above remedies refer to cases of functional emphysema where damage to the alveoli is partial. Structural emphysema where the tone or elasticity of the alveolar wall is completely lost is unlikely to prove responsive to treatment.

3. PNEUMONIA

Inflammation of the lung tissue is not all that common in the cat. Some forms may arise from various virus diseases e.g. viral pneumonitis. Secondary infection due to different bacterial species sometimes arises as a sequel to viral infection.

CLINICAL SIGNS. The cat is seen to be anxious and shows increased respirations; a rise in temperature is commonly seen. There is a general look of unease in the animal and a tendency to stay still. Sternal recumbency is the norm with the mouth open to aid breathing.

TREATMENT

1. ACONITUM. This remedy should be given as early as possible when symptoms are first seen. Suggested potency 10m, giving one dose every hour for 3 doses.

2. ANT TART. A very useful remedy in broncho-pneumonic states where there is an abundance of loose mucus, and expectoration. Suggested potency 30c, giving one dose twice daily for 7 days.

3. BRYONIA. When the animal is obviously better at rest and resents movement this remedy should be considered. Pressure over the chest brings relief. Suggested potency 6c, giving one dose three times daily for 7 days.

4. ARSEN IOD. A useful remedy for the less severe case or one which is of a recurrent nature. The skin is usually dry. Suggested potency 12c, giving one dose twice daily for 7 days.

5. FERRUM PHOSPH. The cat may show signs of pain and anxiety on inspiration. There is an abundance of loose mucus in the throat. Coughing may produce a rusty discharge. Suggested potency 12c, giving one dose three times daily for 5 days.

6. LYCOPODIUM. A useful remedy for the older lean animal showing an exacerbation of symptoms in late afternoon. Suggested potency 12c, giving one dose three times daily for 7 days.

7. *PHOSPHORUS.* Expectoration of blood-stained mucus associated with rapid breathing may be helped by this remedy. Occasionally the cough may be dry and unproductive. This is a useful remedy for nervous and sensitive animals. Suggested potency 30c, giving one dose twice daily for 10 days.

4. PLEURISY

Inflammation of the pleural membranes may be either dry or accompanied by effusion into the pleural sac. It usually arises as a sequel to infection from some part of the respiratory tract.

CLINICAL SIGNS. Anxiety is noticed and abdominal breathing is pronounced. If one side only is affected the animal seeks to lie on that side whereas if the cat assumes a sitting position it usually indicates affection of both sides. A rise in temperature to 105°F occurs. Once effusion into the pleural sac occurs signs of pain diminish.

TREATMENT. The following remedies may be needed depending on overall symptoms:

1. *ACONITUM.* This remedy should always be given early in the condition. A 10m potency should be used, giving one dose every hour for 3 doses.

2. *BELLADONNA.* A useful remedy if the animal feels unduly hot. Showing dilated pupils and nervous symptoms. Suggested potency 200c, giving one dose every hour for 3 doses.

3. *BRYONIA.* This is one of the main remedies to be considered in dry pleuritic cases where the animal is better at rest and resents movement. Pressure over the pleural area gives relief. Suggested potency 6c, giving one dose three times daily for 7 days.

4. *ARSEN ALB.* Older cats may benefit from this remedy especially if symptoms are worse towards midnight and the patient seeks small sips of water. Restlessness is also a feature of this remedy. Suggested potency 30c, giving one dose twice daily for 10 days.

5. PYOTHORAX OR SEPTIC PLEURISY

This term denotes a form of pleurisy accompanied by the production of purulent material in the pleural sac. This condition is seen in cats of all ages and breeds and has been known to occur as a sequel to various viral infections e.g. F.V.R. and Enteritis. Sometimes worm infestation of the lungs predisposes to it.

CLINICAL SIGNS. Occasionally the condition is hyperacute and little or no symptoms are noticed before death. Milder cases show lethargy and depression with indisposition to movement. Increased respirations are noticed. The pulse may become weak and thready. The cat assumes sternal recumbency and assumes this position if made to move.

TREATMENT. The following remedies should be tried:

1. ACONITUM. Should be given as soon as possible as it will relieve stress and anxiety. One dose of 10m should be given and repeated every hour for 3 doses.

2. BRYONIA. This is probably the best remedy to consider when the animal shows signs of umwillingness to move. A guiding sign is relief obtained by pressure over the pleural area. Suggested potency 6c, giving one dose three times daily for 8 days.

3. HEPAR SULPH. The pressence of purulent material in the pleural sac suggests that this remedy may help. Signs of pain may be present in some cases, e.g. on pressure over the area (the opposite of the preceeding remedy). Suggested potency 30c, giving one dose twice daily for 7 days.

4. SILICEA. Milder or long-standing cases may respond to this remedy. It will help resolve any purulent material and will aid the healing of the pleural sac. Suggested potency 200c, giving one dose twice weekly for 4 weeks.

5. PYROGEN. Those cases showing a discrepancy between pulse and temperature e.g. high temperature and weak thready pulse will benefit from this remedy. It is always indicated in septic conditions showing the above discrepancy and also in those cases showing the reverse of such symptoms. Suggested potency 1m, giving one dose every hour for 4 doses.

Diseases of the Nervous System

These are much less common in the cat compared to the dog but occasionally disturbances of function are met with giving rise to varying degrees of neurological involvement. In-coordination of movement, ataxias of different degrees of severity and epileptiform seizures have all been monitored.

1. EPILEPSY

This term encompasses conditions ranging from single fits or black-outs to ongoing seizures which have no regular pattern. Various clinical signs are presented ranging from hyperactivity to loss of consciousness recovery from which shows the animal in a dazed state unresponsive to touch or its surroundings. Thiamine deficiency has been shown to be implicated in many cases of fits when cats are fed on a diet deficient in the substance. Some authorities have considered excess consumption of tinned foods to be a cause in some cases.

TREATMENT. The following remedies will be found useful in controlling the condition in the great majority of cases although it will be found that many animals are resistant to treatment and that the condition itself is extremely unpredictable in nature.

1. BELLADONNA. This is one of the main remedies to consider, indications for its use being unconsciousness, dilated pupils and a throbbing pulse. Suggested potency of 200c to 1m should help, giving a dose hourly for 3 doses.

2. COCCULUS. For long-term cases and fits which come on associated with travel or unusual movement this remedy should prove useful. Suggested potency of 6c given frequently for 3 or 4 doses will help in acute cases. Longer term treatment e.g. daily for 21 days, will help prevent relapses.

3. *CICUTA VIROSA.* The water hemlock remedy is useful for those cases which present with the animal showing unusual neck symptoms e.g. bending the head back or showing a lateral deviation. A potency of 30c will help giving it daily for 10 days.

4. *STRAMONIUM.* A remedy to consider when fits are preceded by the animal falling to one side especially the left. Suggested potency 30c, daily for 7 days.

5. *AGARICUS.* Fits are preceded or followed by incoordination leading to exaggerated stumbling movements (e.g. similar to a drunken gait). Potencies of 6c – 30c twice daily.

6. *PLUMBUM MET.* Many of the heavy metals are associated with brain disturbances of different kinds and this remedy has been used successfully in the treatment of fits where the animal shows weakness of muscles and a bluish-grey appearance of skin and mucous membrances. Suggested potency 30c, daily for 21 days.

7. *CUPRUM MET.* This metal also has proved useful, concomitant symptoms being those of cramping movements and restricted movement. Suggested potency 6c, three times daily for 14 days.

Other remedies which may have to be considered depending on overall symptoms presented are *ABSINTHUM* 6c, *ZINC MET* 30c, *ARNICA* 30c, *NAT SULPH* 200c, *BUFO* 30c, *OPIUM* 30c, and *TARENTULA HISP* 30c. Reference should be made to the Materia Medica for a complete symptom picture of these remedies before deciding on any given one.

2. STROKES

This syndrome sometimes appears in older cats and is thought to have its origins in arterial thrombosis of differing degree.

CLINICAL SIGNS. After initial onset which is invariably sudden, various degrees of immobility may arise e.g. paralysis of facial or head muscles or more extensive paralysis of one side of the body. Mild cases may show little more than incoordination and a tendency to circle to one side or the other. Disturbances of vision may present as a cross-eyed appearance, and a discrepancy in pupils e.g. contraction of one and dilation of the other. Involvement of lip muscles may lead to salivation and drooling.

TREATMENT. There are many useful remedies to consider, chief among which are the following:

1. ACONITUM. The usually sudden onset calls for this remedy initially as it will quickly allay shock and enable other remedies to act more efficaciously. A high potency should be given e.g. 10m, repeated in 30 minutes.

2. OPIUM. This is one of the main remedies for stroke syndrome, where the patient loses consciousness, pupils are constricted and breathing is heavy and stertorous. Recovery is accompanied by excessive drowsiness. Suggested potency 200c, repeated in 2 hours.

3. CONIUM. Conium has a useful action in the older animal. Prominent among its indications are weakness in the hind legs after recovery. Suggested potency 30c daily for 10 days.

4. BUFO. Nose bleeding often accompanies a convulsive attack when this remedy is indicated; these usually give relief. Noise and light aggravate the condition. Prior to an attack the head may be drawn backwards or to one side. Suggested potency 30c, twice daily for 10 days.

5. ARNICA. One should not forget this common remedy in this connection when we consider that a stroke is after all a form of injury. Suggested potency 200c, daily for 3 days.

3. LOCOMOTOR ATAXIA

This condition which presents as posterior weakness of the hind legs and incoordination is occasionally encountered in the older cat. The origin may lie either in a disturbance of the central nervous system or be associated with a lesion somewhere in the spinal cord e.g. affection of a vertebral disc.

CLINICAL SIGNS. A tottering or unsteady gait is evident leading to an inability to ascend stairs or take exercise. Exaggerated movements of varying sorts may be encountered.

TREATMENT. The following remedies should be considered:

1. CONIUM. When hind-limb weakness is prominent this remedy takes pride of place. It strengthens muscle weakness and will make the patient more mobile. Varying potencies may be needed from 30c through to 10m.

2. AGARICUS. Exaggerated stepping movements should be helped by this remedy. The gait has been likened to drunken movements. Staggering is common due to a feeling of dizziness, but there is an absence of convulsions. Suggested potency 30c, daily for 10 days.

3. LATHYRUS. Indications for this remedy are paralyses of varying kinds affecting the motor nerves. It may give results where other remedies seemingly more appropriate have failed e.g. Conium. Potency, 200c, 3 times per week for 4 weeks.

4. CAUSTICUM. A useful remedy for the older cat showing involvement of one particular nerve e.g. sciatic or radial giving rise to a localised paralysis.

5. GELSEMIUM. Mild cases showing a general weakness of the neuro-muscular system may benefit from this remedy. Smaller peripheral nerves are frequently more affected than the larger nerve trunks. Suggested potency 200c, three times weekly for 3 weeks.

4. RADIAL PARALYSIS

Damage to the radial nerve in the fore-limbs is not uncommon in the cat and arises from injury of one kind or another to the nerve at its point of origin in the shoulder or axillary area.

CLINICAL SIGNS. The fore-limb assumes a dropped appearance with consequent knuckling of the foot. This leads to the top area of the foot being dragged along the ground. The general appearance is that of one leg being longer than the other.

TREATMENT. Depending on the degree of damage to the nerve, treatment may be satisfactory or not, and prognosis should be guarded. Slight damage may respond to one or other of the following remedies:

1. PLUMBUM MET. This is probably the most useful remedy to employ to begin with, a successful outcome having been obtained in many cases. Suggested potency 30c, daily for 3 weeks.

2. LATHYRUS. This remedy also has a good reputation in motor paralysis and should be considered if results with the foregoing remedy are indifferent. Suggested potency 200c, three times per week for 4 weeks.

3. CAUSTICUM. More suitable for the older cat presenting a 'run-down' appearance and general weakness. The subject is usually chilly and is susceptible to chilly winds or draughts. Suggested potency 30c, daily for 14 days.

4. GELSEMIUM. Mild cases which may involve accompanying smaller nerves should be helped by this remedy. There is an overall picture of weakness and lassitude. Suggested potency 200c, three times per week for 4 weeks.

5. ANGUSTURA VERA. A lesser known remedy which has an action on the nerves of the lower limbs and feet and should be remembered in this connection as a possible adjunct remedy. Suggested potency 30c, daily for 10 days.

5. MYELITIS

This is the term used to denote inflammation of the substance of the spinal cord. It may be due to infective agents such as specific viruses.

CLINICAL SIGNS. Both motor and sensory nerve tracts may be involved giving rise to a variety of symptoms such as loss of sensation in the limbs and tail or paraplegia in those animals which are severely affected. Alteration to gait arises and there may be loss of control over bladder and bowel functions.

TREATMENT. The following remedies have all been used with varying degrees of success and should give encouraging results in cases which are not too far advanced.

1. CONIUM. This remedy is almost specific for those cases which show hind-leg weakness ranging from slight ataxia to paraplegia where there is a progressive upwards involvement of the disease process. Suggested potencies ranging from 30c – 10m may be needed.

2. LATHYRYS. Indications for this remedy are paralysis of varying kinds affecting especially motor nerves and the remedy is relevant to other areas of the body as well as the hind-limbs. Suggested potency 200c, three times weekly for 4 weeks.

3. GELSEMIUM. Mild cases showing general weakness of various nerve tracts should benefit from this remedy. Lassitude is a common feature. Potencies of 30c – 200c should be considered daily for 10 days and then three times weekly for 3 weeks.

4. SILICEA. If hardening of the nerve sheaths has taken place or is suspected this remedy may help. It is particularly indicated in the treatment of the lean or apparently less well-nourished animal. Suggested potency 200c, 3 times weekly for 6 weeks.

6. DYSOTONOMIA. KEY-GASKELL SYNDROME

This neurological condition of the cat is fortunately less common today that it was a few years ago. The etiology is obscure and the syndrome itself relates to an imbalance of the autonomic nervous system leading to an imbalance of the sympathetic/parasympathetic nerves. The animal presents a picture of dilated pupils with clinical symptoms of difficulty in swallowing due to inactivation of oesophagus together with inactivity of bowel movement.

It is a difficult condition to treat but the following remedies have been known to give some relief in a few cases.

1. GELSEMIUM. 200c given daily for 10 days.

2. OPIUM. 200c given twice weekly for 3 weeks.

3. ATROPINEM. 6c given 3 times daily for 7 days.

Diseases of the
Cardio-Vascular System

1. THE HEART

Abnormalities of heart function are not particularly common in the cat (compared with dogs). Perhaps the most frequently encountered condition is valvular disease or incompetence. The distinguishing signs of this condition may have to be elucidated by professional investigation, outward signs being limited to lethargy and loss of appetite.

TREATMENT. The following remedies have proved of value in valvular heart conditions:

1. LYCOPUS. There is an exaggerated pulse which is quick and irregular. Breathlessness is prominent. Suggested potency 3x, giving one dose twice daily for 30 days.

2. ADONIS. This is one of the best remedies for valvular disease. Urine output is decreased and the urine contains albumen and casts. The heart action is exaggerated. Suggested potency 1x – 2x, giving one dose three times daily for 21 days.

3. CONVALLARIA. The pulse is full and intermittent and the animal is disinclined to move. Suggested potency 2x, giving one dose three times daily for 21 days.

4. LILIUM TIG. The pulse is small and rapid but weak when this remedy is indicated. Even slight movement exacerbates the condition: it sometimes acts better in the female. Suggested potency 3c, giving one dose twice daily for 30 days.

2. ARTERIAL THROMBOSIS

Thrombosis of different parts of the arterial system is not uncommon in the cat. Causation of this problem is somewhat indefinite and it could be due to some inherent abnormality of the blood in any given patient. It frequently comes on suddenly. Very young and very old cats are less susceptible than other age groups.

CLINICAL SIGNS. These vary according to the arterial complex involved, but generally the animal exhibits a collapsed state with signs of pain or discomfort in the area involved. Visible mucous membranes become pale or in severe cases cyanosed. Difficult breathing is pronounced. One of the commoner areas involved is the iliac, producing occlusion of the iliac or femoral vessels. In such cases pulsation of the area is lost. Enlargement of and pain in abdominal muscles is also a feature of this particular form.

TREATMENT. Homoeopathy is able to offer more help in this distressing condition than conventional medicine. Chief among remedies to be considered are the various snake remedies such as:

1. CROTALUS. This remedy has a proven record in helping to resolve thrombosed areas in different species. It should be employed in high potency e.g. 10m and given twice daily for five days. There may be a yellowish discoloration of the skin when this remedy is indicated.

2. BOTHROPS. There may be an accompanying haemorrhage from different orifices when this remedy is indicated. It is more indicated in areas other than those relating to the iliac sphere, e.g. cranial haemorrhage/thrombosis. Suggested potency 200c, giving one dose three times daily for 5 days.

3. LACHESIS. This particular snake venom remedy is indicated when the parts affected assume a purplish or blue appearance and more often confined to the left side of the body. Throat symptoms such as pronounced swelling may be present. Suggested potency 30c, giving one dose twice daily for 10 days.

4. VIPERA. The venom of the yellow viper should be considered when paralysis of affected areas becomes noticeable. Pain over affected area is pronounced. Suggested potency 1m, giving one dose three times per week for 4 weeks.

5. SECALE. This remedy should be considered as a sequel to treatment for iliac or femoral thrombosis as it will encourage a normal blood flow to the legs and feet after the affected area has been cleared. Suggested potency 200c, giving one dose three times per week for 4 weeks.

Diseases of the Urinary Tract

Diseases of the kidney and bladder are encountered frequently especially in the older animal and can take various forms. Both sexes are equally affected. The end result of kidney disease which is unresponsive to treatment is uraemia when the kidney tissue is no longer capable of separating waste products from the blood.

1. INTERSTITIAL NEPHRITIS

(a) Acute Form. This may arise as a sequel to viral infection or be due to bacterial activity.

CLINICAL SIGNS. These can develop quickly and are at first accompanied by lack of appetite and depression. The patient is thirsty and vomiting may take place. Temperature rise is common in the early stages. There is tenderness over the lumbar area and arching of the back is seen. Stiffness of gait is pronounced. Elimination of urine is decreased.

TREATMENT. There are many useful remedies employed in the treatment of this condition and these include the following:

1. ACONITUM. This should always be given in the early stages if possible. It will quickly allay fear and distress which accompanies the condition. Suggested potency 10m, giving one dose every hour for 3 doses.

2. APIS MEL. This is a most useful remedy in acute cases, the animal being thirstless and showing an aversion to heat. It helps promote urination and will bring about a feeling of well-being. Suggested potency 10m, giving one dose every hour for 4 doses.

3. ARSEN ALB. Indications for this remedy are restlessness and drinking of small sips of water. Symptoms are worse towards midnight. Vomiting may be a feature and occasionally loose stools. Suggested potency 1m, giving one dose three times daily for 3 days.

95

4. BELLADONNA. The cat will exhibit signs of central nervous disturbance, with dilated pupils and increased body heat. Output of urine is decreased, and what is passed is reddish-brown. Suggested potency 200c, giving one dose twice daily for 4 days.

5. CANNABIS SATIVA. There is frequent urging with this remedy but little comes. The urine contains mucus, pus and possibly blood. The cat may cry with pain. Suggested potency 30c, giving one dose three times daily for 3 days.

6. CHIMAPHILLA. There is scanty urine which is dark and contains sediment. Symptoms are alleviated by the animal moving about. Suggested potency 30c, giving one dose three times daily for 5 days.

7. BERBERIS VUL. Arching of the back and tenderness over the lumbar area are pronounced when this remedy is considered. Symptoms are worse from movement and the urine is deep yellow, indicating involvement of liver which occurs in the provings of this remedy. Suggested potency 30c, giving one dose three times daily for 7 days.

8. TEREBINTHINAE. Symptoms of uneasiness disappear on movement. Frequent desire is present, the urine containing blood and having a sweetish smell. Suggested potency 200c, giving one dose twice daily for 7 days.

9. URTICA URENS. This remedy helps promote urination and helps elimination of toxic material. There may be accompanying urticarial lesions in the skin. Suggested potency 6x, giving one dose three times daily for 10 days.

10. EEL SERUM. The serum of the eel has a pronounced action on kidney tissue. It is indicated in urinary suppression and helps promote good flow of urine in acute cases, the urine showing increased albumen. Suggested potency 30c, giving one dose three times daily for 3 days.

(b) Chronic Form. This is a progressive condition varying degrees of which are encountered in cats of all species as they get old, especially over 12 years of age.

CLINICAL SIGNS. Progressive loss of weight occurs which is accompanied by stomatitis.

Vomiting and increased thirst. The output of urine is increased, the urine being pale and watery. The specific gravity is low reflecting the retention of solids in the tissues. Dehydration is a constant feature, the coat being harsh and dry. Scattered lesions of eczema are sometimes seen.

TREATMENT. The following are the more prominent remedies to be considered:

1. ARSEN ALB. Should be given when the cat shows excessive dehydration with increased thirst and dry staring coat. Itching of various parts is seen and conditions are exacerbated towards midnight. Suggested potency 30c, giving one dose three times daily for 10 days.

2. CHININUM SULPH. The amount of urine passed is excessive, the urine being pale and very watery, accompanied by a sour smell. Skin rash may be prominent and occasionally abdominal bloating may occur. Suggested potency 6c, giving one dose three times daily for 14 days.

3. COLCHICUM. There is increased urination of dark brown colour accompanying joint stiffness and a disinclination to move. Abdominal flatulence may be pronounced. Suggested potency 30c, giving one dose three times daily for 14 days.

4. NATRUM MUR. Excessive urination and frequency is a keynote of this remedy, often worse during the night. Mouth lesions in the form of superficial ulcers and blisters are often present while hawking and scraping of the throat occurs. This remedy is probably one of the best to be considered as clinical records show that the great majority of cats respond well to various potencies. Suggested potencies 200c, giving one dose three times weekly for 4 weeks, followed by 10m and Cm the same way.

5. MERC CORR. A useful remedy when the increased urination is accompanied by straining with possibly mucous diarrhoea as well. Symptoms are worse in the period from sunset to sunrise. Suggested potency 30, giving one dose three times daily for 7 days.

6. PHOSPHORUS. This remedy has a beneficial effect on the kidney tissue. Output of urine is increased. Small haemorrhages may appear in the gums and vomiting of food and water occurs shortly after ingestion. Suggested potency 30c, giving one dose twice daily for 7 days.

2. PYELONEPHRITIS

This condition may arise when there is any obstruction to the passage of urine which can lead to the presence of blood and pus in the urine. It is sometimes bacterial in origin, a specific organism being responsible. In this case a secondary cystitis may be present. The condition is more frequently encountered in the female. If the case is not too far advanced the following remedies may give good results:

1. HEPAR SULPH. This is one of the main remedies to combat pyogenic infections. Treatment may have to be given with different potencies, starting with 30c daily for 7 days, followed by 200c three times weekly for 4 weeks.

2. MERC CORR. There are usually abdominal symptoms present when this remedy is indicated such as slimy, blood-stained diarrhoea which is worse during the night. The urine and pus assume a greenish tinge. Suggested potency 30c, giving one dose three times daily for 7 days.

3. PAREIRA. Severe straining with discharge of mucus and pus from the urethra may indicate this remedy. There is tenderness over the kidney area. The urine smells strongly and the cat assumes a pronounced crouching attitude when attempting to urinate. Suggested potency 6c, giving one dose three times daily for 10 days.

4. UVA URSI. With this remedy the urine is exceedingly strong and contains whole blood. The urine is dark greenish in colour and straining is again pronounced. Suggested potency 6c, giving one dose daily for 10 days.

5. E. COLI. It sometimes happens that the E. coli organism is responsible for the production of infection in this condition and the use of the nosode is appropriate. A daily dose of 30c for 5 days can safely be combined with any of the foregoing remedies.

3. NEPHROSES

This is the term used to describe degeneration and consequent necrosis of the secreting tubules of the kidney and their obstruction on account of various deposits within them.

Various toxins are usually implicated in the process, chief among which are chemical agents and secondary products from infected wounds or burns.

CLINICAL SIGNS. In the early stages there is marked diminution of urine output and in severe cases where the secreting tubules are blocked with crystalline casts there may be a complete cessation of urination. The early stage is shortly replaced by increased urination which shows blood cells and albumen casts. Diagnosis of this condition depends very much on laboratory urine examination when specific gravity readings and other tests will reveal the exact nature of the problem.

TREATMENT. In this condition emphasis is laid on remedies which have an action on the kidney tissue and have in addition the reputation of being good constitutional remedies. Chief among these are the following:

1. PLUMBUM. This metal in the crude state has a destructive action on kidney tissue and we should therefore expect it to have a beneficial effect in preventing further degeneration when used in potency. There are often accompanying paraplegic tendencies when it is indicated accompanying muscular wasting. Suggested potency 30c, giving one dose twice daily for 14 days.

2. PHOSPHORUS. This element also has a destructive effect on parenchymatous tissue producing a necrosis with accompanying constitutional signs of vomiting and capillary haemorrhages. Suggested potency 30c, giving one dose twice daily for 14 days.

3. SOLIDAGO. This is a useful remedy in the early degenerative stage when the urine contains a thick sediment and is dark brownish-red in colour. Phosphates are present in the urine. A remedy which appear to act better in the male. Suggested potency 6c, giving one dose three times daily for 14 days.

4. THUJA. This is a good constitutional remedy in this condition. The urine is frothy showing a cloudy sediment. The cat exhibits signs of pain by licking the bladder area. Dribbling of urine occurs. Suggested potency 6c, giving one dose three times daily for 14 days.

5. ARSEN ALB. Also a good constitutional remedy for the cat which shows a dehydrated coat with accompanying diarrhoea and skin irritation. Suggested potency 6c, giving one dose three times daily for 10 days.

6. MERC CORR. Animals showing ulcerated skin lesions accompanying a slimy mucous blood-stained diarrhoea will benefit from this remedy. It has a marked action on the kidney parenchyma. Suggested potency 6c, giving one dose three times daily for 10 days.

4. UROLITHIASIS. STONE OR CALCULUS FORMATION

This is a constitutional problem which has as its end product the formation, and subsequent deposit in the renal pelvis and bladder of sabulous or gravel material which eventually coalesces into stones or calculi. They are commonly encountered in the bladder and occur more frequently in the male.

Calculi which are predominantly made up of phosphates usually have their origin in an alkaline urine which can predispose to urinary infection. There are the most commonly encountered, others such as cystine or urate calculi occurring less frequently, and more often in particular breeds because of genetic defects.

CLINICAL SIGNS. The first sign observed is usually the passing of blood and the presence of purulent material in the urine. Depending on the degree of advancement of stone formation there may be passage of thickened urine showing heavy deposits or more frank difficulty in passing urine. Pain in the bladder may occasion the cat to cry out and lick the bladder area. Severe pain and discomfort attends the passage of urine which is voided drop by drop.

TREATMENT. Once large stones have formed the only rational treatment is surgical, but in the early stages when the sabulous material has not coalesced into calculi there are a number of useful remedies available which will prevent further involvement and in many cases dissolve the gravelly material. Chief among these are the following:

1. LYCOPODIUM. This remedy has a tonic action on the liver and will

100

help control the metabolism of that gland, malfunction of which is frequently associated with gravel formation. Cats which require this remedy are in the older age group and invariably are lean and wizened looking. The urine shows a reddish discoloration on standing. Suggested potency 12c, giving one dose twice daily for 21 days.

2. *BERBERIS VUL.* This remedy acts in much the same way as the preceding. Indications for its use are tenderness over the lumbar area and a yellow discoloration of the urine. Suggested potency 12c, giving one dose twice daily for 21 days.

3. *HYDRANGEA.* This is an important remedy which helps both prevent calculi if given as a routine and also aids in the dissolution of gravel material making it easier for the cat to eliminate it. The urine shows white salts alternating with yellow sandy material. Suggested potency 30c, giving one dose daily for 21 days.

4. *EPIGEA REPENS.* Urinary deposits are of the uric acid type when this remedy is indicated. They take the form of a brownish deposit and urination is accompanied by much straining. Suggested potency 6x, giving one dose three times daily for 14 days.

5. *BENZOIC ACID.* This remedy also shows uric acid deposits in its proving but in this case the urine has a strong disagreeable odour with a catarrhal mucous sediment. Suggested potency 6c, giving one dose three times daily for 10 days.

6. *THLASPI BURSA.* Phosphates are in abundance when this remedy is needed. It will quickly dissolve sabulous material and produces salts in urinary deposits of a brick red colour. Suggested potency 6c, giving one dose three times daily for 14 days.

7. *URTICA URENS.* This remedy also thickens the urine by removing the basic salts which are implicated in gravel formation. It helps increase output of urine. There may be an accompanying urticaria of the skin in certain cases. Suggested potency 6x, giving one dose three times daily for 10 days.

8. *CALC PHOSPH.* This is a good constitutional remedy which will regulate the calcium and phosphorus metabolism and thereby help prevent the formation of phosphates. It should be given as a routine remedy in all young animals up to the age of two years. Suggested potency 30c, giving one dose weekly for 8 weeks. It can be safely repeated after intervals of 2 weeks.

9. LITHIUM CARB. This remedy is associated with turbid urine containing a significant amount of mucus and dark brown deposits. Suggested potency 6c, giving one dose three times daily for 14 days.

10. OCIMUM CAN. This remedy is useful once gravel has formed and when the urine shows a bright red colour with a musky odour. On standing there is sediment of brick red colour. Suggested potency 30c, giving one dose daily for 14 days.

11. CALC REN PHOSPH and *CALC REN URIC* can also be given as supplementary remedies to the above. They will help regulate the metabolism when there is a tendency to stone formation. They should be given twice weekly for 8 weeks and repeated from time to time.

5. CYSTITIS

Inflammation of the urinary bladder can affect cats of all ages and breeds and is of common occurrence. It is invariably associated with various bacterial species chief among which are E. coli and Proteus organisms. The condition is presented in both acute and chronic forms.

CLINICAL SIGNS. In the acute form symptons presented are not unlike those associated with viscine or bladder calculi. There is considerable straining, the cat assuming a crouched position. Urine is voided with great difficulty and contains frank blood. The cat usually cries out in pain. There is a temperature rise in the early stages. The distended bladder is readily palpable but care must be exercised in this connection as the bladder wall could early rupture in extreme cases.

The chronic form shows a modification of the above signs and the cat is much less distressed. In the male cat extrusion of the penis may occur. The bladder walls become thickened and again can be palpated externally.

TREATMENT. In the acute condition the following remedies have all proved useful:

1. ACONITUM. Should be given as early as possible as it will allay stress pain and anxiety. 10m potency should be employed, giving one dose every half hour for 5 doses.

2. CANTHARIS. This is probably the most suitable remedy in the acute stage. Straining is severe and any urine passed is heavily blood-stained. Suggested potency 10m, giving one dose three times daily for 3 days.

3. CHIMAPHILLA. Straining is again evident with this remedy but the urine passed contains more purulent material than blood. The urine is dark green and extremely strong. Suggested potency 6c 3 times daily for 5 days.

4. COPAIVA The urine possesses a sweetish smell and has a frothy appearance. In the male animal there may be frequent licking of penal area. Frequent urging is present. Suggested potency 6c 3 times daily for 10 days.

5. CAMPHORA. Urine is voided slowly and is of yellow-green colour on standing there is a reddish sediment. Suggested potency 30c 2 times daily for 5 days.

Chronic Form. This occurs as a sequel to the acute form. The bladder becomes thick and leathery and signs of discomfort are constantly present. Frequent urging with passage of small drops of urine is noted.

TREATMENT. Many of the remedies associated with the acute form are also indicated in the chronic form. In addition the following remedies should be considered.

1. EQUISETUM. Passage of urine does not relieve symptoms of discomfort. Urination is frequent and worse at night. Suggested potency 30c daily for 10 days.

2. EUPATORIUM PURP. This remedy is sometimes associated with calculi and urine of high albumen content. Suggested potency 6c 3 times daily for 14 days.

3. PAREIRA. This remedy will benefit those cases where the bladder musculature has been unduly thickened. There is an ammoniacal smell to the urine; also a heavy mucus sediment. Suggested potency 6c 3 times daily for 14 days.

4. CAUSTICUM. This remedy follows well after Cantharis in the acute stage. The condition takes a recurrent form. Especially useful in the older animal. Suggested potency 30c daily for 14 days.

5. TEREBINTHINAE. A sweetish smell accompanying blood. Stained urine may call for this remedy. Symptoms of discomfort are eased by movement. Suggested potency 200 c 3 times per week for 4 weeks.

6. *UVA URSI*. Signs of pain or discomfort over the entire pubic area accompany the passage of greenish slimy urine which contains blood and purulent material. Passage of urine does not relieve symptoms of pain. Suggested potency 6c 3 times daily for 14 days.

6. HAEMATURIA

The presence of blood in the urine is usually dependent on some disturbance of the urinary tract. Any condition may lead to it and common among these are acute cystitis and lithiasis, but pelvic disease of the kidney may also lead to the presence of blood. Treatment should be directed to the basic disturbance, but the remedy *TEREBINTHINAE* in 200c potency is useful for idiopathic haematuria. Other remedies to consider are *FICUS RELIGIOSA* 6c, *MILLEFOLIUM* 30c and *CROTALUS* 1m.

7. PARALYSIS OF BLADDER

This is usually the result of some injury which has affected the pelvic area leading to loss of function of nerves governing the bladder function. If injury is suspected *ARNICA* 30c should be given first. One dose three times daily for 3 days. This should be followed by *HYPERICUM* 1m, one dose daily for 7 days. The remedy *CONIUM MACULATUM* should be considered in chronic cases as it is a most useful remedy to aid the function of motor nerves.

8. SPRAYING

This distressing complaint is one of the most difficult to deal with involving as it does psychological and emotional disturbances. A thorough investigation of the circumstances surrounding this habit may lead to a remedy which could prove useful if only in a palliative sense. Male cats have been known to spray shortly after the operation for neutering and here the remedy *STAPHISAGRIA* takes pride of place. A dose of 6c three times per day for 7 days should be given and, if necessary, continuation with a higher potency e.g. 200c three times per week for 4 weeks. This remedy is also applicable to the female cat under the same circumstances.

In the male cat also the habit may have its origin in territorial marking and if this is thought likely, the remedy *USTILLAGO MAYDIS* should be considered, giving it in 200c potency three times per week for 4 weeks.

In the neutered animal the accompanying use of the potentised hormones e.g. *FOLLICULINUM*, *OVARIUM*, *OESTROGEN* and *TESTOSTERONE* may also have to be considered. Potencies of 6c to 30c daily for 30 days are usually sufficient to bring about some response, used in conjunction with or after the other remedies mentioned.

The Reproductive System

The autumn period is associated with an abeyance of sexual activity in the cat e.g. October to late December.

The breeding season starting in early January may run for a few months with some cats exhibiting oestrus signs as late as mid-summer. The age at which females show signs of oestrus vary from as early as 4 months to as late as 1 year in individual cases and oestrus may continue into what is relatively middle to old age. The cycle itself lasts roughly three weeks, strong signs lasting about seven days within that period.

1. INFERTILITY

For practical purposes this term refers to the queen and under this heading we can consider those animals which show little or no sexual activity; also those which fail to conceive: and also the care of the queen once she has become pregnant. Queens which show little or no desire may benefit from one or other of the following remedies.

1. SEPIA. This remedy has a beneficial action on the entire female reproductive tract and will regulate hormonal activity in the proper way. It should be used in 200c potency once per week for 3 weeks.

2. PLATINA. This is a remedy which is peculiarly suitable to the Siamese cat as this breed exhibits qualities which are psychologically associated with this remedy. A potency of 30c should be used giving it three times per week for 2 weeks.

If it is thought that ovulation is at fault preventing conception the remedy *PULSATILLA* should prove effective as it has a beneficial action on the ovary, a potency of 30c given three times per week for 4 weeks.

Once the cat has been successfully mated there are two main remedies which will help maintain pregnancy: *1. VIBURNUM OP* and *2. CAULOPHYLLUM.*

The former is the remedy of choice to be given in the first month one dose of 30c twice weekly for four weeks. The latter will regulate pregnancy in the later stages and also help ensure a trouble-free parturition. If however there are difficulties when parturition has started it can safely be given to stimulate uterine contractions e.g. one dose every ½ hour for 4 doses. This should obviate the need for conventional treatment.

One other remedy which helps at this time is *ARNICA* which given a day or two prior to delivery will hasten resolution of tissues and prevent haemorrhage. One dose of 30c three times daily for 2 days should suffice.

POST PARTUM COMPLICATIONS

These include haemorrhage, mastitis and metritis and deficient milk supply.

2. HAEMORRHAGE

This can take many forms and remedies must be used accordingly e.g. if the blood builds up in the uterus and is expelled in a gushing form and builds up again, the remedy to be considered is *IPECACUANHA* 6c giving it every 2 hours for four or five doses. The blood is bright red.

If haemorrhage takes the form of continual dripping, one of the snake venom remedies should be considered e.g. *CROTALUS HORR* or *VIPERA*. Potencies of 12c may be used.

Dark blood may need the remedy *SECALE* 30c while haemorrhage for miscarrage or abortion need the remedy *SABINA* 6c.

3. MASTITIS

Like haemorrhage different forms of mastitis have to be considered ranging from simple inflammation to abscess formation. Early inflammation and swelling should respond to *PHYTOLACCA* in 30c potency, giving it three times daily for 3 days, followed by one dose every second day for 3 doses. If the gland is swollen and hot *BELLADONNA* 6c will help giving it every 2 hours for 5 doses. Excessive hardening of the gland may need *BRYONIA* 30c or *CALC FLUOR* 30c daily for 10 days. Abcess formation accompanied by pain and tenderness should respond to *HEPAR SULPH* given as for phytolacca. Chronic suppurative states with possible fistula development should be treated with *SILICEA* using a 200c potency twice weekly for 6 weeks.

4. METRITIS

Inflammation of the uterus is a serious condition and calls for prompt attention using high potency remedies to achieve the best results, e.g. the remedy *PYROGENIUM* is frequently indicated when there is a discrepancy between pulse and termperature, e.g. high temperature and weak thready pulse or vice versa. *ECHINACEA* is another remedy which like pyrogen is indicated in septic conditions. Lower potencies should be used e.g. 3x and given frequently. Less acute cases showing discharge call for remedies such as *SEPIA*, *PULSATILLA* or *CAULO-PHYLLUM*. *SEPIA* is a most useful remedy when there is post-partum discharge accompanying a mental state of indifference to the kittens, sometimes manifesting as actual attacking of the young. A 30c potency daily for about 5 days will suffice. *PULSATILLA* is more suitable for the gentler animal showing affection and alternation of moods. Discharges are creamy and bland. *CAULOPHYLLUM* is indicated when any discharge becomes chocolate-coloured due to the presence of blood. A 6c potency 3 times daily for 7 days should suffice.

5. LACTATION TETANY

This condition is less common than in the bitch. It usually follows parturition involving large litters, appearing about 3 to 6 weeks after parturition. The cat is usually presented with symptoms of incoordination, with muscular spasms and collapse following. Rapid respirations with dilation of pupils is sometimes seen.

TREATMENT. This is a condition which if possible should be prevented and to this end the remedy *CALC PHOSPH* 30c should be given daily for 10 days following parturition, reducing to 3 times weekly up to 6 weeks. If the condition does develop remedies such as *BELLADONNA* 30c, *MAG PHOSPH* 30c and *CURARE* 30c may be needed depending on symptoms shown e.g. dilated pupils, muscle spasm etc. Incoordination calls for remedies such as *CICUTA*, *STRAMONIUM*, *AGARICUS* and *SULFONAL* depending again on symptoms presented. The remedy picture for these remedies should be studied in the Materia Medica as there are fine dividing lines between each.

6. DEFICIENT MILK

Useful remedies in this connection are *URTICA URENS*, *AGNUS CASTUS* and *USTILAGO MAYDIS*. 30c potencies should be used and given 3 times per day for about 5 days. Much will depend on overall symptoms presented but probably the one most used is Urtica.

7. PYOMETRA

This condition is occasionally seen in the older queen which has not bred for some time.

The condition is presented with the cat showing increased thirst, with vomiting and abdominal distension pronounced. A rise in temperature accompanies a picture of depression and listlessness. In some cases the distended uterus can be palpated. As in the bitch open and closed forms are recognised, the latter being the more common in the cat. If the condition is open the discharge is at first clear and mucoid becoming purulent later due to secondary infection.

TREATMENT. In the open case the following remedies should be considered:

1. HYDRASTIS. Useful in the early stages with clean or mucoid discharge. Suggested potency 30c twice daily for 7 days.

2. PULSATILLA. A suitable remedy for the affectionate animal showing alternation of moods accompanying a bland creamy discharge. Potency 30c, daily for 10 days.

3. SEPIA. Discharges are associated with cats of temperamental disposition with a tendency to attack their kittens or be indifferent to them. Potencies of 6c to 30c should be used three times daily for 7 days.

4. PYROGEN. A most useful remedy when there is a discrepancy between pulse and temperature e.g. high temperature alternating with a weak thready pulse or vice versa. Potencies of 200 to 1m should be used and given 3 to 4 hours apart for 4 doses.

5. CAULOPHYLLUM. Discharges are chocolate coloured due to the presence of blood. This remedy will help drain the uterus and tone up the musculature. It may also help in opening the closed case: potencies of 12c to 30c given 3 times per day for 7 days may be needed.

Footnote. This condition must be carefully monitored especially in the closed case as the cat can quickly become very toxic and surgical intervention may be necessary in very acute forms if remedies fail to change the condition to an open form.

Conditions Affecting the Stud Cat

These are not common but occasionally prostate enlargement is encountered, when remedies such as *SABAL SERRULATA, BARYTA CARB* and *SOLIDAGO* may be needed. Probably the first of these is the better known, but Baryta Carb is more suitable for the old animal. They should be employed in Ø to 3x (Sabal Serr) to 30c (Baryta Carb and Solidago) given twice daily for 21 days.

DIMINISHED LIBIDO

Remedies which should be considered in this connection are:

1. LYCOPODIUM. 30c daily for 21 days. Indicated in animals of lean appearance with a tendency to fickle appetite.

2. *DAMIANA*. This is a well known remedy which helps stimulate libido and should be given 3 times daily for 10 days.

3. *AGNUS CASTUS 6C*. There may be an accompanying prostatic discharge when this remedy is needed. It should be given 3 times daily for 14 days.

Diseases of the Ear

Ear conditions are not uncommon in the cat, chief among them being the following:

1. OTODECTIS MANGE

This condition is frequently met with and is commoner in the younger animal.

CLINICAL SIGNS. Shaking of the ears accompanied by scratching are the main signs early on. Excessive formation of wax takes place in the ear, and the scratching eventually leads to scab formation on the ear flap. Secondary infection leads to a purulent exudate and ulceration of the ear flap.

TREATMENT. External lotions of various kinds are indicated e.g. *CALENDULA Ø* diluted 1/10 and also *HYDROGEN PEROXIDE* diluted 1/3 with warm water. The following remedies will act constitutionally and aid recovery:

1. HEPAR SULPH 30C. Given in the early stages, this remedy will help allay irritation and sensitivity. One dose daily for 14 days.

2. GRAPHITES 6C. If any discharge in the early stages appears as sticky and glutinous this remedy should prove useful. One dose three times daily for 10 days.

3. PSORINUM 30C. Indicated in those cases showing excessive itching accompanied by the animal seeking warmth. One dose daily for 12 days.

4. CINNABAR 12C. This compound of mercury has given good results when other symptoms agree, e.g. worsening of the condition from sunset to sunrise and a tendency for any exudate to become purulent. One dose twice daily for 21 days.

5. MALANDRINUM 200C. This nosode (prepared from grease in

horses) has proved effective in many cases. Two doses a week apart aiding the action of other remedies. Discharges are somewhat like those of *GRAPHITES* but are more glutinous and honey-coloured.

6. *ARSEN IOD 30C.* This remedy may prove useful in the very early stages where symptoms present as a simple imflammation without any noticeable discharge. Dosage one daily for 10 days.

7. *RHUS TOX 1M.* Indicated when the ear flap is also reddened and inflamed accompanying the production of numerous small vesicles. Itching is intense. Restlessness is usually an accompanying symptom. Suggested dosage one daily for 14 days.

8. *TELLURIUM 30C.* Eczematous lesions appear on the outer ear flap when this remedy is indicated. The left ear is more often infected and produces an acrid watery discharge with an offensive smell. Neglected forms may show ulceration of the ear drum with suppurative discharge. Dosage daily for 14 days.

2. OTITIS EXTERNA

This condition is commoner in older cats, and is frequently a sequel to a notoedric infestation.

CLINICAL SIGNS. Shaking and scratching of ears is first seen and this leads on to thickening of the skin which becomes discoloured.

TREATMENT. The following remedies are indicated according to symptoms presented:

1. *SILICEA 30C.* This is a useful remedy when thickening of ear tissue is prominent. It should help control any tendency to suppurative involvement. A daily dose for 14 days should suffice.

2. *TELLURIUM 30C.* Affects the left ear more than the right. This is a good general remedy and should be considered in the more established cases. The ear smells offensive. Daily dosage for 21 days may be needed.

3. *CINNABAR 12C.* If the condition becomes exacerbated from sunset to sunrise this remedy may have to be considered. Other mercury

symptoms may supervene such as salivation and brownish pigmentation of the skin. Dose daily for 14 days.

4. CALC FLUOR 30C. This is a useful tissue remedy and will hasten the healing process. Like *SILICEA* it should help reduce any excess thickening of the integument of the ear. Three times per week for 4 weeks should be tried.

5. PSORINUM 30C. Excessive itching and a tendency for the animal to seek warm places indicates this remedy. The ear smells unpleasant and the animal has a generally unkempt look. Dose daily for 14 days.

3. OTITIS MEDIA

Inflammation of the middle ear structures is not uncommon in the cat and is frequently accompanied by nervous signs. It is frequently bacterial in origin. Pyogenic organisms of various species being implicated.

CLINICAL SIGNS. The owner's attention is first drawn to the animal displaying an abnormality in gait, e.g. staggering to one side, or exhibiting exaggerated limb movements. Moving in a circular fashion may develop and this feature extends also to the head which may be turned around frequently. There may in some cases be a purulent exudate, but this is not a constant sign.

TREATMENT. This may be prolonged and difficult, but the following remedies are all indicated depending on overall symptoms:

1. ACONITUM 30C. Should be given as soon as possible when symptoms first manifest themselves. It will help delay shock and distress. Dosage every hour for 4 doses.

2. STRAMONIUM 30C. When there is a tendency for the animal to fall towards the left side this remedy should prove useful. It should be given daily for 10 days.

3. CICUTA VIROSA 30C. Indicated when there are general head symptoms such as bending the head backwards on the neck or showing an S shaped curve. Dosage one daily for 14 days.

4. AGARICUS 1M. There is a general incoordination of movement when this remedy is needed, giving a 'drunken' picture, e.g. inability to stand properly and exaggerated limb movement. Dosage one daily for 10 days.

5. *MERC SOL CM*. A high potency of this remedy has been found useful in controlling cases showing purulent involvement. A single dose should be given and the resultant response monitored carefully.

6. *HEPAR SULPH 200C*. When the condition is attended by extreme sensitivity to touch indicating pain this remedy may prove useful. In this potency it may help prevent the condition going on to more septic involvement. Daily dosage for 5 days should suffice.

7. *BELLADONNA 200C*. If there is a tendency to central nervous system involvement leading to fits this remedy may be needed. Concomitant features would be dilated pupils and a bounding pulse. A thrice weekly dose for 3 weeks should suffice.

8. The use of nosodes such as *STAPHYLOCOCCUS*, *PASTEURELLA* and *PSEUDOMONAS* should be considered if it is thought that one or other of these organisms is associated with the trouble. A daily dose for 5 days will complement other remedies.

4. AURAL HAEMATOMA

This condition is not uncommon as a sequel to or accompanying other forms of ear trouble. It develops as a result of constant shaking and/or scratching of the ear. It arises because of blood being liberated into the ear between the cartilage and the pinna of the ear. Becoming trapped there the condition presents as an egg-like swelling frequently hot and tender with possible skin discolouration. Normally the fluid part of the blood will be resorbed gradually but there is usually a residual swelling which can persist for some considerable time leading to crumpling of the ear flap.

TREATMENT. Although this is primarily surgical, the following remedies will help the resorption of blood and render any operation that much easier:

1. *ACONITUM 30C*. Should be given as soon as possible helping as it does to allay shock and distress. One dose hourly for 4 hours.

2. ARNICA 30C. As the condition is primarily an injury this remedy is obviously indicated. It aids resorption of blood and will limit damage to the pinna. One dose three times daily for 5 days should be given.

Attention should be directed to the underlying cause, invariably otitis media or externa and the remedies indicated under those headings should be considered.

Diseases of the Eye

These encompass the various eye structures but are less common than in the dog. The eyelids are seldom affected except in some viral conditions of young animals, but occasionally entropion is seen affecting mainly the centre area of the eyelid rather than the corner. This produces lachrymation due to irritation.

Medical treatment is frequently unsatisfactory but the remedy *BORAX* has proved effective in some cases in a potency of 12c, given twice daily for 21 days. Simple lachrymation of unknown origin may respond to remedies such as *BROMIUM 12C*, *ALLIUM CEPA 12X* and *RHUS TOX 1M*.

1. CONJUNCTIVITIS

This condition is not uncommon and is sometimes associated with viral or bacterial infections.

CLINICAL SIGNS. Intense lachrymation is first seen, the discharge being clear to begin with and later becoming brownish and mucoid. Occasionally the third eyelid is protruded, and the condition may be unilateral or bilateral. The latter is usual if the condition is allergic in origin. A deep red appearance of the eye is present.

TREATMENT. The eye should be bathed with a dilute (1/10) solution of *HYPERCAL* (Hypericum and Calendula), once or twice daily and consideration given to one or other of the following remedies:

1. ARGENT NIT. This remedy is a very useful one in alleviating the condition. The animal is usually of a timid disposition exhibiting signs of fear when approached. Suggested potency 30c, giving one dose daily for 7 days.

2. PULSATILLA. This is a suitable remedy for young animals of an affectionate disposition showing changeable moods. Eye discharge tends to become purulent due to secondary infection. Suggested potency 6c, giving one dose three times daily for 7 days.

3. LEDUM. If the condition has arisen as a result of a scratch or stabbing injury to the eye this remedy should be used. Suggested potency 6c, giving one dose three times daily for 7 days.

4. RUTA GRAV. This remedy has a soothing effect on eye structures and will quickly allay pain. Suggested potency 1m, giving one dose daily for 7 days.

5. RHUS TOX. A suitable remedy for bilaterial conjunctivitis arising from allergic causes. There is intense irritation and the eyelids become swollen with possibly loss of hair around the margins. The animal is restless and appears to gain relief by moving from place to place. Suggested potency 1m, giving one dose daily for 10 days.

6. HEPAR SULPH. A remedy which is suited to the acute state showing rapid purulent involvement. There is extreme sensitivity to pain or touch. Suggested potency 1m, giving one dose twice daily for 6 days.

7. ARNICA. This is the obvious remedy if the condition follows mechanical injury of eye structure such as a blow. Suggested potency 6c, giving one dose three times daily for 5 days.

8. MERC SOL. Chronic states which show a worsening of the condition during the night may need this remedy. Eye discharges are greenish in colour and there may be an accompanying stomatitis. Suggested potency 30c, giving one dose three times weekly for 4 weeks.

2. KERATITIS

This is the name given to inflammation of the cornea, and covers also simple erosion and ulceration. In erosion the cornea loses its sheen appearing dull. Lachrymation is usually present to some degree.

Corneal ulceration is not uncommon and is sometimes referred to as ulcerative keratitis. The ulcers may arise as a result of extensive injuries but can arise as a sequel to systemic involvement. They are usually centrally placed and can become subject to secondary infection.

CLINICAL SIGNS. These are usually obvious because of the readily identifiable lesions but in addition there is a strong aversion to light.

TREATMENT

1. ACIDUM NITRIC. This is a useful remedy if superficial ulceration is present. There may be accompanying ulceration around the mouth or nostrils and sometimes loose motions as well. Suggested potency 200c, giving one dose three times weekly for 4 weeks.

2. KALI BICH. This remedy is also associated with ulceration but in this case the ulcers are more deep-seated and have a punched out appearance. There may be an accompanying lachrymation of a yellow colour. Suggested potency 30c, giving one dose daily for 7 days.

3. CANNABIS SATIVA. If corneal opacity is prominent this remedy should give good results. The eye has a generally cloudy look and appears dull. Suggested potency 12c, giving one dose twice daily for 15 days.

4. CALC FLUOR. This remedy also is indicated when opacity is prominent but in this instance there are systemic signs of glandular involvement e.g. swelling of submaxillary or other glands. However as a good tissue remedy it could give good results independent of these signs. Suggested potency 30c, giving one dose three times weekly for 6 weeks.

5. SILICEA. A good remedy for long-standing cases showing scar formation and involvement of the pupil. It will suit animals of lean or wiry formation showing possibly signs of general body weakness. Suggested potency 200c, giving one dose twice weekly for 6 weeks.

6. RUTA GRAV. As in conjunctivitis this remedy will quickly allay pain and general involvement. Suggested potency 1m, giving one dose daily for 10 days.

7. PHOSPHORUS. This is one of the most important remedies to consider in affections of the eye in general. There is usually a bloodshot appearance the cornea showing small red marks or streaks. Suggested potency 30c, giving one dose daily for 10 days.

3. THE UVEA

The vacular layer of the eye which includes the iris, ciliary body and the choroid is referred to as the uvea. Inflammation of any of these structures is referred to as uveitis, chief among which are those affecting the iris and ciliary body (iridocyclitis). This can arise as a sequel to infection from wounds or from extension of a corneal ulcer.

The condition may be acute or chronic, the former showing as increased vascularity with exudation of the iris and ciliary body. The pupils are contracted and there is aversion to light. Exudation of aqueous material which includes white cells gives a clouded appearance to the eye.

More chronic forms exhibit adhesions between the iris and the lens which can lead to glaucoma.

TREATMENT

1. ACONITUM. Should be given as early as possible, a potency of 10m being used and repeated hourly for 3 doses.

2. SYMPHYTUM. This remedy has a beneficial action on the eye structure after injuries and will help allay pain and discomfort. Suggested potency 200c, giving one dose three times weekly for 2 weeks.

3. SILICEA. When adhesions are present as in the more chronic forms this remedy should aid their resorption. Suggested potency 200c, giving one dose twice per week for 6 weeks.

4. HAMAMELIS. When there is marked vascularity involving small venous structures giving the eye a dusky appearance this remedy may help. Suggested potency 12c, giving one dose three times daily for 7 days.

5. PHOSPHORUS. If there is a tendency to glaucoma developing this remedy should be considered. It will also help any ocular haemorrhage. Suggested potency 200c, giving one dose three times weekly for 4 weeks.

4. THE LENS

The main condition affecting this structure is cataract which is less common in the cat than in the dog. It may be congenital or acquired and show different degrees of involvement. Medical treatment if considered should be governed by the use of the following remedies, all of which have been known to have a long term beneficial effect.

1. CALC FLUOR. This is a good constitutional tissue remedy and has helped prevent further deterioration in early stages of the trouble. Suggested potency 30c, giving one dose daily for 14 days.

2. SILICEA. This is one of the main remedies to consider in established cases helping to resorb scar tissue. Suggested potency 200c, giving one dose twice weekly for 8 weeks.

3. NAT MUR. This is a most useful remedy in those cases accompanied by kidney involvement. The patient is usually thirsty and loss of condition is a prominent sign. Suggested potency 30c, giving one dose daily for 21 days.

4. CINERARIA. This remedy should be used in Ø using a dilution of 1/10. It has been shown to be highly beneficial in this condition, adding 2 – 3 drops twice daily for about 2 months.

5. THE RETINA

The conditions which are important in the cat are retinal haemorrhage, retinal detachment and glaucoma which comes into this study.

Retinal haemorrhage is accompanied by dilation of pupils and in severe cases loss of sight. The main remedy in this instance to consider is *PHOSPHORUS* which has given consistently good results. It can be used in various potencies, e.g. 200c three times weekly for 2 weeks, followed by a potency of 1m three times weekly for 4 weeks. Long term therapy should be directed to maintaining the vascular structures in a healthy state and in this connection the snake venom remedies should be considered. Chief among these are *CROTALUS HORRIDUS, BOTH-ROPS LANCEOLATUS* and *VIPERA* all of which help to avoid thrombosis of blood-vessels and thereby will ensure a good blood-supply to the retina. Potencies of 200c given twice weekly for 6 weeks should suffice.

Retinal detachment, although primarily a surgical condition, may react favourably to homoeopathic treatment in mild cases. One clinical case in the author's experience responded well to *PHOSPHORUS* 200c, giving one dose three times weekly for 2 weeks. This was monitored by ophthalmoscopic examination from an independent specialist source, and is mentioned here as an example where homoeopathic treatment should be considered even although the condition is thought to be beyond strictly medical treatment.

6. GLAUCOMA

This condition represents a situation where damage to the retina and optic nerve is brought about by an increase in intraocular pressure due to a build-up of the vitreous humour. It is usually secondary to some other affection of the eye such as uveitis. Acute and chronic congestive forms have been noted, the former showing as reddening of the conjunctiva with a watery discharge with the eye partly shut. Palpation of the eyeball is resented. The cornea becomes severely clouded. The chronic state follows on from the acute in the absence of treatment. The whole eye is greatly enlarged, the blood-vessels being markedly engorged. The cornea may become thickened and possibly ulcerated.

TREATMENT. This can frequently be unrewarding, but the following remedies are worthy of consideration:

1. ACONITUM. This should be given when it will quickly allay pain and stress. A potency of 10m should be used, repeating it hourly for 3 doses.

2. APIS MEL. Considering the build-up of vitreous humour and other fluids this remedy will aid resorption to a certain degree. Suggested potency 30c, giving one dose twice daily for 14 days.

3. BELLADONNA. As there will probably be throbbing and pulsation of vascular structures in the eye this remedy will help. Pupils will be dilated and there may be a state of excitability present. Suggested potency 1m, giving one dose daily for 7 days.

4. SPIGELIA. As pain in the early stages will almost certainly be felt this remedy may help in controlling it; although most of the signs associated with this remedy are subjective these should not inhibit its use. Suggested potency 6c, giving one dose three times daily for 10 days.

5. COLOCYNTHIS. This remedy also comes into the same category as the preceding. In addition there may be abdominal signs such as colic and discomfort. Suggested potency 1m, giving one dose daily for 10 days.

6. *PHOSPHORUS*. In more long-standing cases this remedy should be considered. As mentioned in other instances the remedy has a profound action on the eye structure in general. Suggested potency 200c, giving one dose three times weekly for 4 weeks.

Diseases of Blood and Blood Forming Organs

1. Anaemia

This is the general term given to a diminution in the amount of oxygen in the red cells and any reduction in its circulation causes weakness with pallor of visible mucous membranes. Anaemia can arise as a direct result of loss of blood which could be due to a sudden haemorrhage or to slow bleeding which may be present over a longer period. Parasitical infestations and some infections also give rise to anaemia while disease of the bone-marrow may produce the condition by interfering with the production of blood cells.

(a) ANAEMIA DUE TO ACUTE HAEMORRHAGE. This invariably corrects itself if not too severe and the blood forming organs soon make good the loss of red cells. Remedies which will hasten the coagulation of blood and reduce bleeding include the following, all of which have been well proven:

1. ACONITUM. Indicated for any acute tensive state leading to congestion with fever or inflammation. Such conditions could cause rupture of superficial blood-vessels e.g. in the nose leading to epistaxis. The blood is bright red. Suggested potency 10m, repeated every hour for 3 doses.

2. ARNICA. When haemorrhage is due to the effects of trauma or extreme congestion. Bleeding may take place from any orifice and is due to stasis giving rise to passive haemorrhage of an oozing nature. Blood may be dark. Suggested potency 30c or 200c, repeated every 3 hours for 4 doses.

3. FICUS RELIGIOSA. This is a good general anti-haemorrhage remedy. Vomiting of blood may take place and haemorrhage can occur from any body orifice, the blood being bright red. Suggested potency 6c, repeated frequently.

4. MILLEFOLIUM. The blood again is bright red and associated with acute conditions showing a rise of temperature. The urine may contain blood and haemorrhages can occur from lungs and bowels. Suggested potency 30c, three times daily for 4 days.

5. CROTALUS HORRIDUS. Haemorrhage may be associated with septic states and jaundice but not always. The blood is dark and remains fluid, coagulation frequently being lost entirely. There is a tendency to generalised haemorrhage and the urine becomes dark red. Suggested potency 12c to 200c, repeated three times daily for 5 days.

6. VIPERA. Like other snake venom (with the exception of *NAJA*) this particular one causes passive bleeding with a neurotoxic action in addition. Haemorrhages are often related to the area of lymphatic vessels. Suggested potency 1m, repeated three times per day for 4 days.

7. LACHESIS. This remedy is again associated with conditions which bear a similarity to those brought about by snake-bite. In the particular case of Lachesis there is an accompanying bluish or purplish discoloration of the skin and haemorrhages are dark and passive. Septic involvement is again a feature. Suggested potency 30c, three times daily for 5 days.

8. IPECAC. Haemorrhages are profuse and gushing with bright red blood. It has proved very effective in post-partum bleeding, the blood coming in large gushes instead of a steady stream. There may be associated vomiting and a dislike of food. Bleeding may also occur from the bowel and lungs. Suggested potency 30c, every 2 hours for 5 doses.

9. MELILOTUS. A very useful remedy for haemorrhage from the nose or mouth, the blood being bright red. The blood vessels of the neck and throat are tense and throbbing. There is a general tendency to congestion of the arterial system. Suggested potency 6c, every 2 hours for 5 doses.

10. HAMAMELIS. This is a useful remedy for controlling haemorrhages associated with passive congestion of the venous system. The blood is dark. Suggested potency 30c, three times daily for 5 days.

11. PHOSPHORUS. A most important remedy when there are small capillary haemorrhages in various areas, especially from the gums. Vomiting of blood-stained material may take place and also coughing of rust-coloured sputum. Suggested potency 30c, three times daily for 7 days.

(b) ANAEMIA ASSOCIATED WITH DISTURBANCES OF THE HAEMOPOIETIC SYSTEM. Bone marrow disease which produces pernicious anaemia in man is uncommon in the cat and such disturbance in this species is referred to as aplastic anaemia. It is invariably associated with toxins or severe infections of the chronic nature, e.g. it has been known to arise as a result of over-prescribing of certain powerful drugs. It may also be associated with vitamin deficiency and it is good practice to administer organic vitamin supplements e.g. vitamin E and those of the B complex.

CLINICAL SIGNS. These are similar to those of anaemia in general.

TREATMENT

1. TRINITROTOLUENE. There may be an accompanying toxic jaundice present when this remedy is indicated. It is an extremely useful remedy in restoring the power of the haemoglobin to transport oxygen. There are also present weak heart beats, increased respirations and high-coloured urine. Suggested potency 30c, twice weekly for 14 days.

2. SILICEA. This is a remedy to consider if it is thought that the condition has arisen as a result of long-standing infections. It is a valuable remedy also if the anaemia accompanies general malnutrition and has a specific action on bone disorders. Suggested potency 200c, twice weekly for 8 weeks.

3. ARSEN ALB. This deeply acting remedy will aid those cases showing extreme weakness and exhaustion with accompanying restlessness and thirst for small amounts of water. It has a valuable reputation in the treatment of chronic anaemia. Suggested potency 1m, daily for 21 days.

4. MERC SOL. Mercury produces severe anaemia and is a remedy which should be considered when the specific accompanying symptoms are present e.g. excess salivation and slimy diarrhoea with skin eruptions. Suggested potency 6c, three times daily for 10 days.

5. CINCHONA. This is homoeopathic quinine and is a prime remedy for any condition resulting in weakness due to loss of vital body fluids. Suggested potency 6c, three times daily for 7 days.

In all cases of suspected anaemia the animal's blood should be subjected to a proper laboratory examination. This will determine the type of anaemia present and whether there is in addition a corresponding imbalance in the leucocyte (white cell) count which could indicate some accompanying disorder.

Allergic Conditions

1. ANAPHYLAXIS

This is the term used to denote a hypersensitive state which can be brought on by contact with some specific antigen or by the cat receiving antibodies from another animal, e.g. by serum injection. Also certain tissues may contain substances which are conducive to an anaphylactic attack.

CLINICAL SIGNS. It may present as a local or widespread inflammatory process ranging from arteriole contraction with circulatory weakness to the onset of severe functional states. Anaphylactic shock is frequently attended by vomiting, diarrhoea and severe prostration and as a rule arises quickly after exposure to the antigen concerned, usually hyperimmune serum. Other signs include difficult breathing, loss of balance and paleness of visible mucous membranes.

TREATMENT. If it is possible to supply aid in time, the following remedies may help:

1. ACONITUM. This remedy should be given immediately as it will help combat shock especially in cases which show suddenness of onset. Suggested potency — a single dose of 10m should suffice.

2. CAMPHORA. This is a very useful remedy for collapsed states showing diarrhoea and extreme coldness of body surfaces. Stools are watery and dark and attacks of diarrhoea come on suddenly. Suggested potency 30c, repeated frequently.

3. CARBO VEG. When signs of air hunger or dyspnoea appear, this remedy will benefit the patient. It has a sound reputation for giving strength and warmth to apparently moribund states. Suggested potency 200, repeated as necessary.

4. VERATRUM ALB. This remedy is also useful in cases of collapse with prostration and diarrhoea, but unlike the Camphor picture, symptoms are less severe. Stools tend to be greenish. Suggested potency 30c, every 3 hours for 4 doses.

5. *RESCUE REMEDY*. The Bach Flower Remedies are not potentised but are extremely useful in many conditions. This particular one is most helpful in combating physical or mental trauma and promotes a feeling of well being.

2. ALLERGIC CONTACT DERMATITIS

This is the term used for those cases of hypersensitivity — often delayed — when the animal shows a reaction to an agent which contacts the skin, such agent being of an irritating nature. Exposure to the particular agent may be short or prolonged depending on the agent involved. The animal must have a predisposition to the condition.

CLINICAL SIGNS. Lesions are usually confined to the hairless parts such as the inner legs, inguinal area and the interdigital spaces. Erythematous swellings at first develop which later become papular. Severe cases will include most parts of the body.

TREATMENT. The following remedies should be considered:

1. RHUS TOX. Indicated for the early erythematous stage before papules develop. Itching may be severe. Suggested potency 1m, repeated every hour for 3 doses.

2. ANTIMONIUM CRUDUM. A useful remedy for the papular stage of the lesion and will help prevent development of vesicles. Suggested potency 6c, three times daily for 3 days.

3. THALLIUM ACETAS. A useful remedy to promote healthy functioning of skin after other remedies have aided the healing process. Suggested potency 30c, daily for 7 days.

6. MIXED GRASSES. This remedy has been developed to help those cases which arise as a result of contact with spring grasses. Suggested potency 30c, daily for 10 days.

5. CORTISONE 30c, *BETAMETHASONE* 30c and *PREDNISOLONE* 30c. These potentised steriods have proved useful in their own ways in controlling the inflammatory process without producing any side-effects. They should be given daily for 7 days.

6. SPECIFIC NOSODE. Made from the agent responsible. It should be

129

used in 30c potency and can be combined with other indicated remedies.

3. CAR SICKNESS

This distressing condition is fortunately less common in the cat than in the dog but occasionally is met with. Under this heading we can consider any motion which brings about symptoms of discomfort to the animal experiencing travel, and includes air and sea-sickness as well as the much commoner car sickness.

CLINICAL SIGNS. Signs of distress soon become apparent after transportation beings and include panting, salivation and vomiting. Sometimes bowel evacuation takes place also. Signs of inappetance and distress may continue for some little time after the journey has finished and are probably accompanied by nausea as in the human subject.

TREATMENT. Animals should not be subjected to car or air journeys immediately after a meal. It is a good plan to keep the cat basket on the floor of the vehicle where the animal cannot see out of the window as visual disturbances are thought to play a part in the onset of symptoms. The main remedy to consider is *COCCULUS* in either *6c or 30c* potency, giving a dose or two shortly before the journey commences. Other remedies which have also helped are *PETROLEUM 30c* as the smell of petrol fumes appears to upset some cats. *TABACUM 30c* especially useful for sickness associated with sea travel. *IPECAC 30c* where vomiting is frequent and accompanied by signs of nausea. *APOMORPHINE HYDROCHLORIDE 6c* where severe and persistent vomiting supervenes accompanied by much salivation.

Diseases of Muscles

1. MYOSITIS

Inflammation of muscle fibres is sometimes met with, although less frequently encountered than in dogs.

ETIOLOGY. The cause may be either systemic or traumatic. If the origin is systemic there is usually a bacterial or viral infection present while trauma is associated with injury of one kind or another. Traumatic lesions usually lead to septic involvement of tissues which can be extensive in some cases.

CLINICAL SIGNS. There may be swelling of the particular muscle but frequently no special signs are evident and the owner's attention is drawn to the fact that the animal cries out on being moved or lifted. Various postures are assumed according to the muscles affected e.g. arching of the back when the lumbar muscles are involved. A board-like feeling of the abdomen indicates pain of the muscles of that region.

TREATMENT
1. ACONITUM. This should always be considered in the early stages as it will bring about relief from pain, especially if the origin is bacterial or viral. It will allay any tendency to shock if the condition arises suddenly. Suggested potency 1m, hourly for 3 doses.

2. RHUS TOX. This remedy is indicated when the animal gains relief from movement even although the initial movement is painful. It may influence the muscles of the left side of the body more than the right and is indicated when severe wetting or prolonged damp is associated with the onset of symptoms. Suggested potency 6c, twice daily for 21 days.

3. BRYONIA. Movement is resented when Bryonia is indicated. The animal will seek to lie on the affected muscle and pressure on it gives relief. Warmth is appreciated also. Suggested potency 6c, twice daily for 15 days.

4. CURARE. This remedy is indicated when there is a generalised muscular weakness present or a state of semi-paralysis arises. Muscular reflexes are abolished. Suggested potency 30c, daily for 14 days.

5. CAUSTICUM. When there is an accompanying contraction of tendons and stiffness of muscles this remedy may help. Warmth again brings relief. The remedy is more adaptable to the older patient showing unsteadiness of gait. Suggested potency 12c, twice a day for 14 days.

6. ZINC MET. This remedy is associated with trembling of affected muscles. The condition usually follows bacterial or viral infection. Suggested potency 30c, daily for 21 days.

7. STRYCHNINUM. Indicated when severe contractions of muscles take place as part of an overall systemic involvement and various postures may be seen. Suggested potency 30c, daily for 15 days.

8. GELSEMIUM. Weakness and a tendency to paralysis is the keynote of this remedy. There may be a generalised involvement of all muscles and the trouble is usually systemic in origin. Exercise may lead to collapse. Suggested potency 12c, daily for 14 days.

2. PANSTEATIS. YELLOW FAT DISEASES

This condition implies a condition which can arise from an unbalanced diet which is preponderantly that of fish of one kind or another, particularly those which are rich in oils. It is relatively uncommon but may be encountered from time to time.

CLINICAL SIGNS. The animal resents handling and there is an appearance of lethargy with disinclination to move. Loss of appetite is common together with a rise in temperature. Abdominal palpation is resented and small lumps of fat may be palpated.

TREATMENT. Excess fish should be eliminated from the diet, and the following remedies considered:

1. BRYONIA. This remedy is indicated as most cases appear to be better when at rest. Suggested potency 6c, three times daily for 3 days.

2. ACONITUM. Should be given early if there is a temperature rise.

132

This will stabilise the temperature and allay any tendency to shock. Suggested potency 1m, hourly for 4 doses.

3. NUX VOM. Inappetance should be relieved by the use of this remedy and appetite thereby stimulated. Suggested potency 6c, three times daily for 5 days.

4. CALC FLUOR. This remedy should help dispel any small lumps of fats which have developed. Suggested potency 6c, three times daily for 7 days.

5. SILICEA. If the condition has become chronic and there is a tendency for fat lumps to become firm, this remedy should help. Suggested potency 200c, twice per week for 6 weeks.

Diseases of Musculo-Skeletal System

A. BONE DISORDERS AND DISEASES

These are relatively uncommon in the cat but occasionally one or other of the following conditions may be encountered:

1. OSTEOPOROSIS

This term is used to describe the condition in which bone becomes increasingly porous. It is due to metabolic upsets which result in a deficiency of bone formation and may follow systemic disease of varying kinds. The animal may show an increased tendency to fractures.

TREATMENT. The following remedies may all prove useful:

1. CALC PHOSPH. This is a very useful remedy for the younger animal in the growing stage as it exerts a profound influence on the development of bone and muscle. Suggested potency 30c, daily for 21 days.

2. CALCAREA FLUOR. The fluoride of calcium is a good tissue remedy and is instrumental in hardening bone and strengthening the periosteum. Suggested potency 30c, daily for 21 days.

3. HECLA LAVA. This remedy also exerts an action on bone producing in the crude state exostoses of varying kinds, excess of which leads to brittleness and fractures. Homoeopathically it gives good results in such cases. Suggested potency 12c, twice daily for 21 days, followed by 1m once weekly for 4 weeks.

4. SILICEA. This is also a good tissue remedy exerting a beneficial action on the skeletal system in general. Suggested potency 200, once weekly for 6 weeks.

2. OSTEOMYELITIS

This term refers to an infection of bone which, in the acute form, has its origin in the cavity of bone known as the medullary cavity. A more chronic form originates in the periosteum and leads to the formation of sinuses opening on the skin.

ETIOLOGY. The acute form arises when pyogenic bacteria gain entrance to the medulla of the bone either through blood transfer or via compound fractures. Chronic osteomyelitis can develop when infections reach the periosteum and can follow punctured wounds or bites. The main pyogenic organisms which are associated with this condition are Staphylococci and to a lesser extent Streptococci.

CLINICAL SIGNS. Acute disease is characterised by lameness, febrile attacks and swelling of the affected limb. Sinus formation with purulent discharge is often the early sign of the chronic form and febrile signs are much less evident.

TREATMENT. The following remedies are useful in controlling both the acute and chronic forms:

1. ACONITUM. Should always be given in the early febrile stage of the acute stage. It may have to be repeated for one or two doses. Suggested potency 1m, hourly for 4 doses.

2. HEPAR SULPH. In the acute form accompanying severe pain this could prove a very useful remedy, a guiding symptom for its use is extreme sensitivity to pain. Suggested potency 30c, three times daily for 7 days.

3. RUTA GRAV. This remedy has a beneficial action on infections or inflammations of the periosteum and should therefore prove beneficial in the acute form which may thus prevent the more chronic form arising. Suggested potency 6c, 3 times daily for 10 days.

4. CALC FLUOR. This remedy should prove useful in the treatment of the young animal in the developing stage. Suggested potency 30c, three times per week for 6 weeks.

5. SILICEA. A suitable remedy for the chronic form where sinuses have formed. Suggested potency 200c, twice weekly for 6 weeks.

6. TUB BOV. Although this condition is not thought to be associated with tuberculosis as in many cases in the human being it is nevertheless worth keeping in mind as a useful remedy in controlling bone affection of this nature. Suggested potency 200c, once monthly for 3 months.

7. SYMPHYTUM. A useful remedy to consider when there is a tendency for bone to weaken or fracture. It is a good general healing agent. Suggested potency 200c, once weekly for 8 weeks.

8. STAPHYLOCOCCUS AUREUS. This nosode should be combined with selected remedies. A single dose of 200c should suffice.

3. RICKETS AND OSTEOMALACIA

These terms denote a failure of bone to assimilate minerals such as calcium and phosphorus, leading to softening of bone and distortion and thickening of joints. The term rickets is used to describe the condition in the young growing animal while the other relates to the same condition in the adult animal.

ETIOLOGY. The basic cause is failure of the calcium/phosphorus metabolism and its relation to Vitamin D resulting in a deficiency of the latter.

CLINICAL SIGNS. The softening of the bones in rickets produces a bowed appearance of the limbs while enlargement of the joints at the end of the bones leads to painful swellings. These appear as 'bead-like' protuberances where the ribs are involved. Early involvement produces severe lameness. Osteomalacia is less associated with bone distortion and lameness is the predominant symptom.

TREATMENT

(a) Rickets. While the condition is relatively uncommon in the cat the following remedies should be kept in mind:

1. CALC PHOSPH. The main remedy to consider as it will help stabilise the calcium/phosphorus ratio. Suggested potency 30c, twice weekly for 6 weeks.

2. CALC CARB. This similar remedy may be needed if results are not encouraging with the previous remedy. It is more suitable for kittens of the Persian and Birman breeds.

(b) Osteomalacia. SILICEA, HECLA LAVA and CALC FLUOR are all useful remedies to help strengthen bone. Potencies ranging from 12c to 200c may be needed.

5. OSTEOGENESIS IMPERFECTA

This condition in the cat is of more common occurrence than the former ones and may appear as a result of animals being subjected to a calcium deficient diet. Some authorities consider the Siamese breed to be peculiarly susceptible.

CLINICAL SIGNS. The kitten appears less active than one would expect. Brittleness of bone leads to spontaneous fracture preceded by extreme pain and lameness. X-ray examination may be necessary in obscure cases.

TREATMENT. Calcium and phosphorus are the two elements which are concerned and should be employed as CALC PHOSPH 30c, giving it twice weekly for 8 weeks. HECLA LAVA will help strengthen bone in those cases showing early brittleness and should be employed in 12c potency twice weekly for 4 weeks. SILICEA is a remedy to consider for more long term use, a potency of 200c being useful twice weekly for 6 weeks.

5. TUMOURS OF BONE

These comprise osteosarcomas of different types and are occasionally met with. They may develop in different areas, but most commonly in the upper forelimb and upper hind-limb. They are presented as swellings of differing degrees and are usually accompanied by pain and lameness. They are difficult to treat, but success has attended the occasional case by using remedies such as SILICEA, HECLA LAVA, CONDURANGO and CALC FLUOR in potencies of 30c–200c.

137

6. ARTHRITIS

Of the two forms of arthritis encountered viz. osteoarthritis and rheumatoid, the latter is possibly more commonly seen. Osteoarthritis affects mainly the spinal vertebrae resulting in a form of spondylitis. The animal shows lameness and a disinclination to move. Manipulation of joints is resented. Remedies to consider are *RHUS TOX* in 6c to 1m potency, *BRYONIA* in 6c potency, *ACID SAL* 30c, *ACTAEA RAC* 30c, *MINERAL EXTRACT* 6x. Treatment may have to be given over a long period, alternating the remedies according to response.

In so-called rheumatoid arthritis there are different joints involved, very rarely a single one. The smaller joints e.g. carpus (wrist) are more often affected, and accompany an increase in joint fluid which causes painful swelling.

CLINICAL SIGNS. include a rise in temperature and severe pain on manipulation of joints. Loss of appetite accompanies malaise and weight loss.

TREATMENT. Remedies such as *RHUS TOX* (6c–1m), *ACID FORMIC* (6c), *ACTAEA RAC* (30c) and *CAULOPHYLLUM* (30c) have all proved useful according to overall symptoms. *APIS* (30c) is also indicated if there is an excess of synovial fluid causing puffy joint swellings.

7. EXCESS OF DIETARY VITAMIN A

The feeding of too much liver has been shown in the cat to result in bony enlargements of certain joints, especially carpus and neck region. In several cases complete absence of joint movement may occur. Loss of movement results in wasting of muscles involved. Any treatment to be successful must depend on discontinuing liver as a source of food and substituting it with protein of a different nature e.g. kidney. If the condition has not advanced too far, remedies such as *RHUS TOX* (6c–1m), *ACID SAL* (30c), *CAULOPHYLLUM* (30c) and *ACTAEA RAC* (30c) are all worthy of consideration. Mild cases may resolve spontaneously if the liver diet is discontinued.

Miliary Eczema and Alopecia

Both these conditions occur in cats of both sexes as a result of neutering, symptoms appearing at variable intervals after the operation. It is common in the female and presents as a less serious problem than in the male.

CLINICAL SIGNS. In the eczema type the animal may show a pimply rash on various areas, particularly along the back and around the head and neck. Alopecia may show as denuded areas of hair along the flank and down the inside of the thighs. Scratching may or may not be present. The animal is usually unsettled and out of sorts.

TREATMENT. The first remedy to consider after the operation for neutering is *STAPHISAGRIA*, which has the virtue of acting on a psychological level helping to remove any feelings of injustice on the part of the patient. This is well documented in the human being so it is reasonable to assume that animals will suffer the same emotions. At any rate it will be found that the remedy in this connection is highly effective. A thrice daily dose of 6c for 3 days should be sufficient.

Remedies for the longer term include the ovarian hormones *FOLLICULINUM* and *OVARIUM* in the female and testosterone in the male. Folliculinum should be given first, a twice daily dose of 6c for 21 days, followed by the same remedy in 30c potency, three times per week for 4 weeks after an interval of one week. In the great majority of cases this regime will give good results. Ovarium acts in a similar way but experience has shown that the results using this remedy are less satisfactory than those obtained with Folliculinum. As this condition tends to recur after a variable interval the procedure may have to be repeated. It will be found in practice that some cats retain the effect of the remedies longer than others.

TESTOSTERONE 30c and 6c may also be used for miliary eczema and alopecia in the male cat following the same regime, but results tend to be less satisfactory than when the female hormones are used.

1. NOTOEDRIC MANGE

This type of mange is not uncommon in the cat and appears mainly on the area below the ears covering the skin towards the eyes.

CLINICAL SIGNS. Mild cases are accompanied by thinning of hair and slight irritation is evidenced by the animal pawing or 'washing' the affected area. More severe forms show an extension of the lesions to the ear and these may ultimately spread down the neck towards the shoulders. The skin eventually becomes thickened and the animal is affected severely by pruritus.

TREATMENT. The following remedies may all prove useful depending on the stage of involvement:

1. MORGAN 30C. This bowel nosode is useful in the early stages and should be given daily for 5 days.

2. SUPLHUR 200C. This follows the previous remedy well and should be given weekly, one dose for 4 weeks.

3. PSORINUM 30C. Indications for this remedy are a desire for warmth (as opposed to Sulphur which seeks coolness) and also excessive pruritis. Dosage is one daily for 14 days.

4. ARSEN ALB 30C. The animal may show systemic involvement such as vomiting and loose stools if this remedy is needed. It is a very useful skin remedy in general. Dose daily for 14 days.

5. THALLIUM ACETAS 30C. This remedy has a trophic action on hair follicles and will help regenerate hair growth provided the follicles have not been destroyed. It is useful after other emergency remedies have been given. Dose daily for 21 days.

6. LYCOPODIUM 200C. This is another useful remedy in mild cases of hair loss or thinning and may be needed when digestive symptoms such as biliousness or liver symptoms are present. Dosage twice weekly for 5 weeks.

Homoeopathic treatment may have to be accompanied by external dressings of suitable type. These should not interfere with remedies if carefully used.

2. RODENT ULCER

This not uncommon skin lesion takes the form of a granuloma which has an unfortunate propensity to become invasive. It occurs on the area above the lip near the junction of skin and mucous membrane.

CLINICAL SIGNS. These are obvious and take the form of an ulcerated area with a concave appearance, and raised edges which proliferate outwards.

TREATMENT. Some animals respond to treatment satisfactorily but others can be refractory. The following remedies have all proved useful:

1. ACIDUM NITRICUM 200C. This remedy is always worthy of consideration in those lesions showing involvement of skin and mucous membrane together. A dose three times per week for 4 weeks should be given.

2. KALI BICH 200C. This is another remedy which has given good results in invasive ulcerative states and many cases of rodent ulcer have responded well to it. One dose three times per week for 6 weeks may be needed.

3. ANTHRACINUM 200C. This nosode in its provings gives a picture not unlike that presented in some rodent ulcer cases where the centre of the lesion becomes necrotic. Two doses of 200c potency a week apart should be tried.

Wounds and Injuries

Any injury or contusion arising without breaking of the skin should be treated immediately with the remedy *ARNICA* using a 30c potency three times daily for 5 days. This will allay any development of more serious involvement arising as a result of the injury. Even although the initial injury was sustained many months before, this remedy will still be indicated. It is particularly effective in soft tissue injuries, e.g. muscles and eyes and will hasten resorption of subcutaneous haemorrhage. Injuries to bone resulting in damage to the periosteum may need the remedy *RUTA* in preference to *ARNICA*, as this remedy has a pronounced action on the periosteal covering. It is also extrememly useful in external injuries to the eyeball e.g. contusions and may safely be given along with *ARNICA* in this respect. The remedy *HAMEMELIS* is also extremely useful in eye contusions and will help along with these other remedies: it will aid the clearance of any blood-shot appearance.

When wounds or injuries are of an open nature involving cutting of skin and involvement of deeper structures, different remedies are called for, chief among which are the following:

1. CALENDULA combined with *HYPERCAL* and any open wounds should be bathed frequently with a solution of the Ø diluted 1/10. This will quickly allay the pain of any nerve involvement. *HYPERICUM 1m* should also be given internally at the same time, a daily dose for 5 days being sufficient.

2. LEDUM. This remedy is most useful when the injury takes the form of a punctured wound e.g. a sting or bite. Combined with *HYPERICUM* it will prevent more serious trouble from arising. Potencies range from 6c to 200 and can be given three times daily for 2 days.

3. HEPAR SULPH. If wounds develop to a suppurative stage as is common in cat injuries this remedy should aid recovery. Given in low potency e.g. 6c it will help promote suppuration and thus aid the healing process in this way. Higher potencies e.g. 200 to 1M will help dry up the process and aid rapid healing. Wounds which need this remedy are accompanied by extreme sensitivity to pain.

4. SILICEA. If the infection of an open wound proceeds to a more chronic stage leading to tissue being under-run with the establishment of sinuses and fistula (a common occurrence in the cat) this remedy should prove useful. Potency of 200c should be considered three times weekly for 4 weeks.

Any injury which involves fractures of bone should benefit from the remedy *SYMPHYTUM* in 200c potency, twice weekly for 8 weeks as an aid to union of fracture. Needless to say this does not take the place of surgical interference, but will lessen the period of convalescence in such cases.

Before leaving the subject of injuries there are two areas of the body which respond to specific remedies which appear to act better than the more recognised remedy such as *ARNICA*: These are injuries to the head and to the coccyx area of the lower spinal column. The former injury responds well to the remedy *NATRUM SULPH* in 200c potency. Any condition developing from a head injury should be treated to begin with by this remedy. The latter injury calls for the use of the remedy *HYPERICUM* in 1m potency, daily for 7 days. This would appear to be as near as possible a specific remedy for this particular type of injury, although one never likes to use the word 'specific' in relation to homoepathic remedies.

Parasites

1. FLEAS

The vexed question of how to combat fleas is one which frequently arises in some animals. Not all cats will become infested and the healthier the animal is and the better fed the less likely such an animal succumbs to infestation. A regular course of *SULPHUR* 30c, twice per week for 4 weeks, and repeated after intervals of 2 weeks without treatment may help to render the animal less attractive to infestation. The use of aromatic oils brushed into the fur twice weekly is also beneficial but as these are very strong-smelling substances their use should be restricted to animals not undergoing homoeopathic treatment. Regular grooming with comb and brush will be helpful. The use of noxious sprays should be avoided at all times. Athough they appear to be effective at the time their use results in a strain of fleas which becomes resistant. The same may be said for flea collars which are again in many cases toxic.

Vaccination Procedure

This is based on the use of nosodes and/or oral vaccines. There is no hard and fast rule concerning frequency of administration but a system which has yielded satisfactory results is to give a single dose (powder or tablet) night and morning for 3 days followed by one per week for 4 weeks and continuing thereafter with a monthly dose for 6 months.

There is a fundamental difference between conventional vaccination by injection and that using the oral route. The former involves the subcutaneous or intramuscular injection of an antigen (vaccine material) which after an interval produces antibodies in the blood-stream against the particular antigen. While in most cases by this method, a degree of protection against the particular disease is established, the procedure can be criticised on two grounds. 1, The defence system of the body is not fully incorporated by this means and 2, there is a risk of side effects due to the foreign nature of the protein involved in the vaccine material. This aspect of conventional vaccination has been well documented in many species.

Oral vaccination on the other hand gives a more solid immunity inasmuch as it incorporates the entire defence system, which is mobilised as soon as the vaccine is taken into the mouth and builds up protection with each further dose. This build up leads on from tonsillar tissue through the lymphatics incorporating the entire reticulo-endothelial system. This procedure is equivalent to what is known as 'street infection' viz. ingestion of virus etc. during daily contact with other animals, when immunity would be built up in the same way.

Manufacturers of conventional vaccines against F.V.R. recognise this principle in marketing a product for use by intra-nasal insufflation.

Another advantage in protection by homoeopathic means is that vaccination can be started very early in the kitten's life e.g. within the first week if necessary. This does not interfere with the presence of any maternal antibodies.

Footnote. The undesirable side-effects which sometimes follow conventional vaccination can in some measure be offset by the use of the potentised virus using ascending potencies at varying intervals depending on the severity of the case. Fortunately as far as the cat population is concerned side effects from conventional vaccination are much less common compared with those occurring in the dog.

There are no side effects when using homoeopathic oral vaccines — a reaction may sometimes be observed, as also occasionally with remedies but such reaction is transient and soon passes.

Specific Diseases

RESPIRATORY VIRUSES

The incidence of respiratory viruses in cats is in direct proportion to the number of cats which congregate in any given area or situation. Spread to other cats rapidly develops when an infected member of a cat 'colony' is brought into contact with isolated individuals. The main viruses which affect the respiratory system are F.V.R. and Fev (Calici).

1. FELINE VIRAL RHINOTRACHEITIS

SYMPTOMS. There is an incubation period of up to 10 days when evidence of conjunctival involvement is apparent leading to a clear discharge. Upper respiratory symptoms show as sneezing and nasal discharge. Temperature may rise to 105°F in severe cases. Salivation occassionally occurs with inflammatory lesions on the throat. At this stage the clearer discharges may become purulent. The disease may proceed to a chronic form when symptoms of bronchitis develop with possibly pneumonia as a secondary complication. Ulceration of the nasal septum affects many cats suffering from chronic infection when the patient may sneeze blood-stained mucus. This ulceration may lead on to necrosis of nasal cartilages and turbinate bones. The disease is most severe in animals at the extremes of life e.g. young kittens and old animals which previously led a sheltered existence. Cats which show a clinical recovery may remain carriers and shed virus under conditions of stress, and may also succumb to the occasional relapse when symptoms again become manifest.

TREATMENT. The following remedies have all proved useful according to sumptoms displayed.

1. PULSATILLA. This remedy has been described as the nearest one can get to a constitutional remedy for the cat, while many cats do indeed

147

respond well to it there are other remedies in this connection which are equally valid. The cat which may be in need of Pulsatilla is usually an affectionate animal showing variable symptoms and alteration of moods. Discharges are usually copious and bland. It is worth considering in the early stages of F.V.R. infection and if the response is good will help prevent any deterioration of the condition leading to chronic involvement. Suggested potency 30c, giving one dose 3 times daily for 5 days.

2. *SILICEA*. If treatment is delayed and secondary involvement of eye structures develop e.g. keratitis this remedy may help. It will speed the resolution of early scar tissue and remove the cloudiness and opacity which apparent in this phase of the disease. Suggested potency 200c, giving one dose three times weekly for 6 weeks.

3. *ANT TART*. This remedy should prove useful if broncho-pneumonic symptoms develop. Coughing is of the moist type and expectoration is muco-purulent, although scanty. The patient in need of this remedy may frequently be seen lying on its right side as opposed to the left. Suggested potency 30c, giving one dose daily for 10 days.

4. *PHOSPHORUS*. This deep acting remedy may be needed when involvement of the nasal septum and turbinate bones develops. Caries or necrosis of these structures calls for this remedy associated with violent sneezing of blood-stained purulent mucus. It may also be indicated in bronchial conditions when the patient coughs up blood-stained mucus. Haemorrhage is a keynote of this remedy along with its destructive effect on various body systems. Suggested potency 200c, giving one dose 3 times weekly for 4 weeks.

5. *KALI BICH*. When this remedy is indicated the nasal and bronchial secretions are thick, tough and yellowish. Expectoration and sneezing show little frank mucus. The remedy is indicated when ulceration of nasal septum develops. Suggested potency 200c, giving one dose twice weekly for 6 weeks.

6. *ACID FLUOR*. Indicated in chronic involvement of nasal septum, especially in the older subject. Pressure over the sinus area is resented. Discharges are offensive and the subject shows a periodicity in its relation to the condition e.g. there may be spells of relief from symptoms alternating with periods when aggravation occurs. Suggested potency 30c, giving 1 dose daily for 14 days.

7. KREOSOTUM. If severe involvement of bronchial structures is suspected or diagnosed leading to the possible development of bronchiectasis the use of this remedy may be indicated. It has frequently been used successfully in this connection. There is a tendency to gangrenous involvement of structures. Breath is extremely fetid. Suggested potency 200c, giving one dose 3 times weekly for 6 weeks.

8. F.V.R. NOSODE. The use of the nosode is always indicated along with selected remedies. This will complement their action and help speed recovery. Suggested potency 30c, giving one dose daily for 7 days.

2. CALICI VIRUS DISEASE

This viral disease shows as a variety of symptoms depending on the severity of the infection and the structures or body systems involved.

SYMPTOMS. Mouth involvement is extremely common presenting as ulceration of tongue and buccal mucosa. The nasal septum becomes ulcerated leading to bouts of muco-purulent sneezing. Pneumonia is a common complication and death is not infrequent in hyperacute cases. Temperature may rise to 105°F. Salivation is profuse, large strings of saliva being seen.

TREATMENT. The upper respiratory system may call for remedies which are indicated for F.V.R. (which see). Others include:

1. MERC SOL. This remedy is indicated when salivation is excessive. It will have a beneficial action on the mouth generally although seldom indicated when ulceration is present. There is a general dirty look to the mouth and the patient is worse from sunset to sunrise. Suggested potency 30c, giving one dose daily for 14 days.

2. BORAX. This is a useful remedy to consider when involvement of oral mucous membranes is accompanied by ulceration. Nervous symptoms develop, the patient showing fear under certain conditions.

There is a strong aversion to descending stairs or jumping from chairs etc. Salivation is again excessive and there may also be tenderness of foot pads. Suggested potency 6c, giving one dose 3 times daily for 14 days.

3. PHOSPHORUS. This remedy should prove helpful when pneumonia supervenes. There is usually rapid involvement of lung tissue with severe difficulty in breathing. Expectoration is scanty and is blood-stained. There may be involvement of liver when this remedy is indicated, bilious vomiting being a feature. Water and food is rejected shortly after ingestion and stools are pasty or clay-coloured. Suggested potency 200c, giving one dose twice weekly for 6 weeks.

4. NOSODE. The use of the nosode is again indicated along with selected remedies, a dose of once daily for 7 days usually sufficing.

3. CHLAMYDIAL INFECTION. FELINE PNEUMONITIS

This disease is associated with a causative agent called Chlamydia psittaci and is becoming more frequent in its distribution spreading slowly among the cat population where previously it was more regional in its distribution involving fewer animals.

SYMPTOMS. The upper respiratory and lachrymal systems are involved leading to rhinitis of an acrid nature. Eye symptoms are prominent conjunctivitis being severe. This produces a gummy sticky discharge which leads to the eyelids sometimes sticking together. Inflammation of the eyelids shows as thickening. Temperature is invariably normal. The condition can be particularly severe in young kittens.

TREATMENT

1. ARGENTUM NIT. A most useful remedy for conjunctival involvement when the inner canthi becomes red and swollen. Purulent involvement is common. Chronic cases may show corneal ulceration and this remedy will help in cases like this. Animals in need of this remedy may show fear of handling manifested by trembling and a desire to escape. Suggested potency 30c, giving one dose daily for 10 days.

2. *HIPPOZAENIUM*. A remedy to consider in rhinitis states when the discharge becomes honey-coloured and sticky. It may be associated with ulceration of the nasal septum. Suggested potency 30c, giving one dose daily for 7 days.

3. *GRAPHITES*. Stickiness of discharges is a keynote of this remedy and is therefore indicated when this feature is prominent especially as regards eye discharges. Severe involvement leading to closure of eyes with sticky discharge calls for the remedy. Suggested potency 6c, giving one dose three times daily for 7 days.

4. *KALI BICH*. Nasal discharges are thick, muco-purulent and yellow, and difficult to expel. Suggested potency 200c, giving one dose twice weekly for 4 weeks.

5. *LEMNA MINOR*. Another useful remedy for nasal discharge showing evil smelling dirty secretions. The patient is sensitive to damp surroundings. Suggested potency 30c, giving one dose daily for 10 days.

6. *ACID NIT*. If corneal ulceration develops this remedy may play a part, especially if the ulceration is near the margin of the eyelids. Bowel symptoms may supervene in the form of colitis producing loose stools of a slimy dysenteric nature. Rhinitis also features prominently in the provings of this remedy and it should be considered in chronic ulcerative states of the nasal septum leading to discharges of a yellow corrosive character. Suggested potency 200c, giving one dose twice weekly for 4 weeks.

7. *PHOSPHORUS*. A deep acting remedy to consider if deeper structures of the eye become involved e.g. iritis and retinitis. It has a profound action on the eyes and also on nasal structures e.g. turbinate bones leading to ulceration and discharge of a purulent nature streaked with blood. Suggested potency 200c, giving one dose twice weekly for 6 weeks.

8. *NOSODE*. A Chlamydia nosode is available which can be used in conjunction with selected remedies. Suggested potency 30c, giving one dose daily for 10 days.

4. FELINE ENTERITIS (PANLEUCOPAENIA)

This is a viral disease caused by an organism of the parvovirus group, manifesting itself as an acute infection which may last up to one week. Morbidity among affected cats is high and mortality rate can be as high as 90% in unprotected animals. It is possible that some animals possess an in-built resistance to the disease.

SYMPTOMS. After an incubation period which may extend to 10 days an affected cat may present in the form of an animal suffering severe colic, viz. arched back, stretching of hind-legs and exhibiting signs of abdominal pain causing it to cry out. Severe vomiting supervenes causing rapid dehydration, and loss of condition quickly sets in, these together producing a desire for water which the patient finds difficulty in lapping. Temperature may rise to 106°F, and the animal presents a hide-bound appearance with sunken eyes and anxious expression. Sternal recumbency becomes a feature as the disease progresses.

TREATMENT

1. ARSEN ALB. The picture of a cat suffering from acute panleuco-paenia represents in most respects a picture of arsenic poisoning with the proviso that in feline enteritis diarrhoea is not always present. It will be seen therefore that Arsen Alb is the remedy of choice to start with. This should help relieve the pain and vomiting and allay anxiety and restlessness. It should be given frequently e.g. every hour for 4 doses using a potency of 1m.

2. ACONITUM. This remedy should be given as early as possible when it will help allay shock and fear and help generally calm the animal. A single dose of 10m potency should suffice.

3. PHOSPHORUS. If vomiting persists after the administration of Arsenicum has been completed this remedy may be needed, especially if improvement has been such that the animal will lap water or milk and then have it rejected shortly afterwards. If there is a tendency for pneumonia to develop as happens in some instances this remedy will again be of great benefit. Suggested potency 30c, giving one dose twice daily for 7 days.

4. BAPTISIA. The post-mortem changes of congested intestinal mucosa, together with haemorrhage suggests that this remedy may also

152

be needed in refractory cases i.e. in those which do not respond well to the previous remedies. There is sometimes a dusky hue to the oral mucous membranes if Baptisia is to be considered. Cats which may react to the disease in an atypical way e.g. suffering diarrhoea are more likely to need this remedy.

5. *CINCHONA (CHINA)*. This remedy should always be considered when treating cases of dehydration and others showing weakness after loss of body fluids. It can be used in conjunction with other remedies and given frequently. Suggested potency 6c, giving one dose 2 hourly for 4 or 5 doses.

6. *PYROGEN*. This is a most important remedy to consider in septic conditions which show a discrepancy between pulse and temperature, e.g. a high temperature alternating with a weak thready pulse as is seen in many cases of panleucopaenia. It will quickly stabilise both pulse and temperature and help induce a feeling of relief in the patient. It should always be used in high potency, e.g. 1m, giving one dose every hour for 5 doses.

7. *CANTHARIS*. The intestinal inflammation which quickly builds up in this disease may produce an accompanying peritonitis when the clinical symptoms of board-like hardness of the abdominal musculature will be evident producing severe pain on pressure over the affected area. Suggested potency 1m, giving one dose every hour for 4 doses. Repeated next day giving one dose 3 times in the day.

PROPHYLAXIS. A nosode prepared from infected material is available as is also an oral vaccine prepared from the virus. For dosage details see introductory chapter on vaccination procedure.

5. CEREBELLAR ATAXIA

The virus associated with this particular condition is closely allied to that which causes panleucopaenia, some authorities considering them to be the same. The virus attacks young kittens producing a picture of motor inco-ordination, unsteadiness of gait, loss of balance and various forms of central nervous system derangement occur. Sometimes there are exaggerated stepping movements while involvement of cranial nerves may lead to difficulty in eating or lapping of water/milk.

TREATMENT. There are several remedies which could prove useful provided destruction of brain tissue has not taken place. Purely functional states may respond.

1. STRAMONIUM. Indications for this remedy are inco-ordination of gait with a tendency to fall on the left side. Clinical cases which show mystagmus (squinting) may also benefit. Eyes wide open and staring. Suggested potency 12c, giving one dose 3 times a day for 7 days.

2. CICUTA VIROSA. The animal may show a tendency to fall backwards when cicuta is indicated, occasionally showing also an S-shaped curvature of the neck. Convulsions could also benefit if there is a disposition to these. Suggested potency 30c, giving one dose twice daily for 7 days.

3. HYOSCYAMUS. Frequent head shaking and a tendency to muscular twitchings accompany abdominal discomfort. The patient may shift from place to place. Suggested potency 200c, giving one dose daily for 7 days.

6. CUPRUM ACETICUM. Involvement of the tongue may be noticed when this remedy is indicated. There may be involuntary twitching movements, the patient putting the tongue in and out frequently. Tenseness and the passage of brown slimy stools may accompany the nervous symptoms. Suggested potency 6c, giving one dose three times daily for 7 days.

5. HELLEBORUS NIGER. Signs of head pains are associated with this remedy; the cat may bang its head against any object in an attempt to obtain relief. Suggested potency 6c, giving one dose three times daily for 5 days.

6. ZINC MET. Rolling of the head is a common symptom together with paddling movements of the feet. The patient is easily startled leading to an exacerbation of symptoms. Suggested potency 30c, giving one dose daily for 7 days.

7. BRYONIA. One should consider this remedy if the cat appears to be better when lying still and movements bring on symptoms of distress, e.g. vertigo when made to rise or move. Desire for water is seen, even although attempts to drink may be unsatisfactory. Suggested potency 6c, giving one dose three times daily for 5 days.

8. SULFONAL. Signs of vertigo appear. Eyes bloodshot, urine scanty and desire frequent: tendency to paralysis. Suggested potency 6c, giving one dose three times daily for 10 days.

PROPHYLAXIS. A nosode prepared from infected material is available as is also an oral vaccine prepared from the virus. For dosage details see introductory chapter on vaccination procedure.

6. ULCERATIVE GLOSSITIS

This is a viral condition affecting mainly young cats although very young kittens are seldom affected. Outbreaks of this disease are usually sporadic in nature and tend not to become widespread.

CLINICAL SYMPTOMS. There is an initial rise of temperature of about 2 – 3 degrees accompanying loss of appetite. Within a few hours salivation appears producing long ropy strands of clear fluid, occasionally viscid, after an initial stage of frothiness. Mucous membranes of mouth and tongue become congested leading eventually to ulceration, seen particularly along the edges of the tongue and spreading over the surface. Severe cases show ulceration as far back as the throat, ulcerative patches tending to vary in size and distribution. Lesions are mostly confined to the mouth and the cat shows little distress apart from the difficulty in eating and drinking during the active phase of the disease.

TREATMENT

1. MERC SOL. This is one of the main remedies to consider in cases of salivation, the ropy saliva being a guiding symptom for its use. There is generally a dirty look to the mouth. Suggested potency 6c, giving one dose three times daily for 7 days.

2. MERC CORR. This remedy should be considered when the case presented shows more severe symptoms than with the previous remedy. Salivation is again prominent, but the degree of inflammation suggests more systemic involvement e.g. dysenteric mucoid stools. Suggested potency 30c, giving one dose twice daily for 5 days.

3. BORAX. A useful remedy when ulceration is the most prominent feature e.g. of the epithelium of the tongue and gums. Salivation is also present and there may be signs of tenderness of the feet, indicated by the animal licking its paws. Fear of downward motion figures prominently in the provings of this remedy which may point to its selection over other competing remedies. Suggested potency 6c, giving one dose three times daily for 10 days.

4. MERC IOD RUB. The double iodide of mercury has an action on the gums and is indicated when the inflammatory process is worse on the left side. Suggested potency 30c, giving one dose twice daily for 6 days.

5. MERC IOD FLAV. Also useful in gingivitis but tends to favour the right side. Both these iodides have given good results in many cases. Suggested potency 30c, giving one dose twice daily for 6 days.

6. MERC CYAN. The cyanide of mercury should be considered when there is severe inflammation of the throat and surrounding glands. The ulcers are surrounded by a greyish membrane. Prostration is a feature of this remedy. Suggested potency 30c daily for 7 days.

PROPHYLAXIS. A nosode could be made from infected material e.g. saliva or associated glands in a clinical case, and thereafter potentised to 30c and administered as with other nosodes/vaccines.

7. FELINE INFECTIOUS ANAEMIA

This is a protozoal disease caused by a blood parasite belonging to the family Rickettsia, and transmitted by insect vectors e.g. blood-sucking fleas. There is also a belief that infection can be transmitted via the placenta. The organisms once established in the host cause destruction of red cells with resultant anaemia.

SYMPTOMS. Occasionally these are somewhat ill-defined, the cat being presented because of general weakness along with loss of appetite. The disease may run a course of 3 weeks to one month. The general signs of anaemia are obvious in established cases e.g. pallor of mucous membranes, lethargy and possibly jaundice. In severe cases there may be involvement of the spleen which becomes swollen and palpable.

Diagnosis may have to depend on blood examination to differentiate the condition from non-specific anaemia, but not every case will show the parasites to be present.

TREATMENT. Protozoal diseases in general are difficult to treat homoeopathically and remedies should be selected on the basis of supportive therapy.

These include:

1. ARSEN ALB. which may help the damage done to the red cells. The increase in leucocytes shown by blood examination is a strong indication for this remedy. Suggested potency 1m, giving one dose daily for 14 days.

2. CROTALUS HORR. This snake venom in potency may be beneficial in those cases showing jaundice. The skin may appear brownish-yellow and blotchy. It is a powerful remedy against conditions resulting in haemolysis (destruction of blood cells) and has a strong haemorrhagic affinity. Suggested potency 200c, giving one dose three times weekly for 4 weeks.

3. LACHESIS. Somewhat similar in its action to the previous remedy, but there is less liver involvement and skin assumes a purplish appearance rather than yellow-brown. Destruction of blood cells again figures in the pathogenesis. Suggested potency 30c, giving one dose twice daily for 10 days.

4. CINCHONA. As in other conditions where weakness and lethargy appear due to loss of essential body fluid, this remedy is indicated as a supplement to other selected remedies. Suggested potency 6c, giving one dose four times daily for 2 days. Can safely be repeated.

8. FELINE LEUKAEMIA FeLV INFECTION

The incidence of this disease is widespread among colonies of cats although not every cat harbouring the virus will necessarily show clinical symptoms. Isolated individual cats are much less at risk. The

157

virus attacks the reticulo-endothelial system which is widespread throughout the connective tissues of the body and therefore is liable to produce disease symptoms and lesions e.g. lymphosarcoma tumours, in various areas.

The virus has a predilection for lymphoid tissue, other body systems being less at risk. although the lymphatic system is mainly involved excretion of virus takes place via other channels, e.g. saliva, milk and urine.

If we imagine different colonies of cats it can be determined that one group or colony harbours neither virus nor antibody and this would represent cats resistant to infection. Because of genetic involvement another colony might represent disease free animals possessing antibodies to infection but not harbouring virus. These animals have proved resistant to infection. A disease free colony would be represented by cats which harbour both virus and antibody. Cats which are at risk and which will probably succumb to infection harbour virus but have no antibodies to the virus.

CLINICAL SYMPTOMS. A variety of clinical signs may be present because of the widespread involvement throughout the reticulo-endothelial system. The virus possesses immunosuppressive properties which leads to the development of disease entities which would not otherwise appear. These may take many forms. Leukaemia and/or lymphosarcoma tumours are the main signs to look out for. Breeding queens may experience abortion or resorption of foetuses with or without vaginal discharge. The immunosuppressive aspect of this disease implies that relatively trivial illnesses may assume more serious proportions because of the body's inability to provide proper protection. The increasing number of nephritis cases among cats presented to clinics and surgeries throughout the country is thought by some workers to be due to the presence of FeLV infection. Anaemia is a prominent symptom and may appear independent of leukaemia. The latter is dependent on disease of the bone narrow releasing malignant cells into the general circulation. Various body symptoms throughout the reticulo-endothelial system become involved leading to the development of the lymphosarcomatous tumours. These may co-exist with leukaemia cases or be independent of them and can occur in mesenteric lymph glands leading to palpable tumours or to breathing problems when the lymphoid tissues of the thymus gland become involved. Tumours of the liver are not uncommon and again may be large enough to be palpated.

DIAGNOSIS. This depends on specific tests available for the identification of the virus, although clinical symptoms are significant to those who have experience of the disease. Sample blood tests are not always reliable.

TREATMENT. Because of the immunosuppressive aspects of this virus, treatment even by homoeopathy tends to be speculative, considering that homoeopathic remedies act through the defence system. A nosode against FeLV is available prepared from a lymphosarcoma tumour and has proved useful in some cases, while other cases have proved resistant to the same approach. Depending upon the body system involved, supportive treatment (combined with nosode) may help. One particular Abyssinian cat with a lymphosarcoma tumour of the liver responded to a combination of nosode and *PHOSPHORUS*, regression being gradual over a period of four months. Multiple involvement of lymph glands is usually refractory to treatment although every effort should be made to alleviate, using selected remedies and nosode e.g. Calcarea Fluorica or Silicea.

PROPHYLAXIS. At the present stage no conventional vaccine is available to combat this disease. A homoeopathic nosode has been prepared from two different sources, one from a lymphosarcoma tumour and two from viraemic blood.

One medicated powder of 30c potency given night and morning for 3 days, followed by one per week for 4 weeks and continued monthly for a further six doses may go some way to limit the development of clinical symptoms in cats which are at risk. (Author's experience)

9. FELINE INFECTIOUS PERITONITIS

This disease which invariably produces fatal peritonitis has recently shown an increase in its distribution. It affects mainly young cats particularly the so-called exotic breeds, although all breeds are susceptible.

CLINICAL SYMPTOMS. After an incubation period up to 14 days or longer, cats may be presented showing an initial temperature up to 106°F. The main sign is abdominal distension due to fluid resulting from a fibrinous peritonitis. Jaundice may be present suggesting liver involvement, while general abdominal discomfort is evident. The pleura may become affected in some cases leading to the production of fibrinous fluid in the pleural sac. This results in difficult breathing.

TREATMENT. This is rarely satisfactory mainly because the condition is terminal when presented. In milder cases supportive treatment may ease the animal's discomfort.

Remedies which have been used in this connection include *CANTHARIS* — always a useful remedy to consider in peritoneal cases, *CARDUUS MAR* for its action on the liver leading to the production of abdominal fluid and *TUB BOV*. The last named remedy is mentioned because of the similarity clinically to abdominal tuberculosis of the bovine which was prevalent in the days before eradication of this disease was undertaken. This produced a peritonitis clinically resembling F.I.P. and the use of the nosode is a logical step to try.

PROPHYLAXIS. A nosode against F.I.P. has been prepared from infected peritoneal fluid and is available for protection using it in the manner suggested for FeLV.

10. TUBERCULOSIS

This disease is much less common today, since eradication of tuberculosis from dairy cattle has removed the main source of infection. Of the two strains of the causal organism Mycobacterium tub. human and bovine, the latter is the one to which cats are most susceptible. There are no particular symptoms indicative of the disease in cats and infection could take many forms, especially disease of bones and glands. Recurrent sinuses and fistulae which shown little tendency to heal should be regarded with suspicion.

TREATMENT is not generally recommended, but if insisted on, the use of the nosode *TUB BOV* may help along with constitutional remedies.

Good feeding and housing are essential. The nosode should be used in the 200c potency, giving a dose per week for 4 weeks. This may have to be repeated after a lapse of 3 months or so.

11. HEPATIC RENAL SYNDROME

This is a condition of indeterminate etiology which affects cats of mainly younger age groups. Owners seek advice because the cats show signs of abdominal discomfort with vomiting and thirst.

CLINICAL SIGNS. On examination, temperature may be as high as 104.5°F while visible mucous membranes show jaundice. If stools are passed, the faeces are characteristically orange-yellow, indicating liver involvement. The kidney may be palpable and urine if passed is highly coloured.

TREATMENT. There are many useful remedies to be considered in this condition, chief among them being:

1. ACONITUM. Should be given early when symptoms first appear. One dose every hour for 3 doses. Suggested potency 1m.

2. PHOSPHORUS. Indications for this remedy include vomiting after food or water become warm in the stomach. A most useful liver remedy. Suggested potency 30c, giving one dose twice daily for 5 days.

3. CHELIDONIUM. Indicated when the syndrome includes jaundice. There may be an accompanying stiffness over the right shoulder area. Suggested potency 30c, giving one dose twice daily for 7 days.

4. CHIONANTHUS. Jaundice is also present when this remedy may be indicated. Stools are clay-coloured: spleen also enlarged. Urine is dark with a high specific gravity. Suggested potency 3x – 6x, giving one dose three times daily for 7 days.

5. CARDUUS MAR. This is a useful remedy when cirrhosis is threatened. There is often an accompanying state of abdominal fluid present. Suggested potency 30c, giving one dose daily for 14 days.

6. LYCOPODIUM. A useful remedy for the older subject, especially lean animals showing hardness of stools. There is a periodicity with this remedy, symptoms being worse in late afternoon. Suggested potency 200, giving one dose daily for 7 days.

6. BERBERIS. This remedy will hasten liver function and will have a beneficial action on the kidneys. Weakness over loins may be seen. Suggested potency 30c, giving one dose daily for 14 days.

8. PTELEA. This is a clearing remedy and will hasten the elimination of waste products from the system. Suggested potency 6c, giving one dose three times daily for 14 days.

12. CRYPTOCOCCOSIS

This is a rare disease of cats which produces granulomatous masses in various areas of the head e.g. nasal passages and around the eyes. Lung complications have also been reported.

TREATMENT is not recommended as there is a possibility that the condition could be transmissible to man in whom it can be extremely serious.

13. TETANUS

Cats, unlike some other species are fairly resistant to infection by the causal organism Cl. tetani. Cases which have been recorded have arisen as a result of wound infection e.g. following surgical interference, bites from rats or other animals and deep puncturing from nails or other sharp objects.

CLINICAL SIGNS. The cat appears on examination to show an increased awareness to sound and to be more susceptible to touch which produces exaggerated muscle movement. Muscles become stiff and a generalised rigidity sets in. In contrast to the disease in other animals the muscles of the jaw do not become fixed (lockjaw) in the great majority of cases. Protrusion of the third eyelid may occur.

TREATMENT

1. ACONITUM. Should be given as early as possible. Three doses of 1m one hour apart.

2. LEDUM. This is the main remedy to consider when a punctured wound has been sustained. Suggested potency 6c, giving one dose three times daily for 4 days.

3. HYPERICUM. This remedy will relieve nerve pain in the wounded area and help limit the absorption of toxin. It combines well with *LEDUM* and should be given in 1m potency daily for 7 days.

4. CURARE. Muscular stiffness and rigidity may need this remedy, with a strong tendency to paralysis: muscles of jaw are affected leading to trismus (lockjaw). Suggested potency 6c, giving one dose three times daily for 10 days.

5. STRYCHNINUM. This remedy should help control the tetanic spasms which sometimes appear in serious cases. Also indicated in those cases where extension and rigidity of limbs appear. Suggested potency 200c, giving one dose daily for 7 days.

6. NOSODE. The use of the nosode in 30c potency will complement the use of the other remedies.

14. TOXOPLASMOSIS

This is a protozoal disease which can infect cats with little or no relevant symptoms appearing. Cats can harbour the parasite and excretion can be a source of danger to man and other animals.

CLINICAL SIGNS. The lymphatic system is again heavily involved, lymphoid tissue here and there being subject to enlargement by granulomatous masses. Lesions of bronchial lymph nodes may lead to pneumonia-like symptoms. Because of the all-embracing nature of the lymphatic system lesions could develop in other areas e.g. kidney and liver.

TREATMENT. This is purely symptomatic based on the reaction of the patient to the infection. *CALC FLUOR* and *SILICEA* are remedies which may prove beneficial, potencies of 30–200c being given at regular intervals e.g. twice monthly for 6 months. A nosode exists which can be used along with selected remedies. Vaccination procedure using the nosode should follow the rules laid down for other diseases.

15. FELINE LYMPHOTROPHIC LENTIVIRUS (FTLV)

This syndrome in cats which has recently been investigated bears a close resemblance to AIDS in the human being. It is considered unlikely that infection could be passed from infected cats. Not all cats which harbour this virus will produce clinical signs even although a latent infection may persist in the system.

Contact among cats in colonies leads to transmission of virus; carrier cats co-exist with clinically infected animals.

CLINICAL SIGNS. The syndrome pursues a chronic course leading to progressive loss of weight and inappetance. Pathological manifestations include gingivitis, skin diseases and rhino/conjunctivitis. Involvement of the lympathic system leads to enlargement of lymph glands. Because of the compromising nature of this virus in relation to the immune system almost any clinical sign may become manifest due to the inability of the body to ward off superimposed infections.

TREATMENT. Inasmuch as homoeopathic remedies act through the immune/defence system, treatment will at best be speculative. However any remedies employed should be related to the overall picture presented, reference being made to the Materia Medica for remedies which could be applicable. The use of a nosode prepared from infected blood or infected material should materially assist the action of selected remedies.

16. RINGWORM

This is a fungal condition affecting the skin and its appendages i.e. hair and whiskers. The epidermis is involved but seldom the subcutaneous tissues. However the latter can be affected in an inflammatory manner leading to a condition called cellulitis.

CAUSATION. The fungal agents called MICROSPORUM and TRI-CHOPHYTON are responsible for both acute and chronic forms. The former is more likely to be encountered in kittens and the latter in older animals.

CLINICAL SIGNS. Scaling of superficial epithelial cells takes place with possibly a serous exudation. Hair loss supervenes leading to areas of depilation particularly around the head, tail and along the back. Less frequently the groin area is affected.

TREATMENT. This can prove to be difficult but the following remedies should be considered:

1. SEPIA. This remedy has a beneficial action on the skin which presents as a scaly dry denuded area. It shoulld be given in 200c potency once per week for four weeks.

2. BACILLINUM. This nosode has proved efficacious in the treatment of ringworm in other species and although its action on cats is less certain it may be worth trying in 200c potency one per week for four weeks.

3. MICROSPORON and TRICHOPHYTON NOSODES. These can be combined and given once per week for six weeks in 30c potency. They will complement the action of other remedies.

Externally the parts should be thoroughly cleaned and treated daily with HYPERCAL lotion diluted 1/10.

17. WORMING

There are remedies that might be considered for cats including Filix mas 3 ×, Granatum 3 × and Kamala 3 ×. These are all useful remedies for the treatment of tapeworm and should be given twice daily for 30 days.

Roundworm infestation is helped by the remedy Chenopodium 3 × and also by Granatum 3 × in the same dosages as for tapeworm.

Index

Abdominal Muscles, Enlargement of
94, 100
Abies Canadensis (Hemlock Spruce)
9
Abortion 107, 158
Abrotanum (Southernwood) 9
Absinthum (Wormwood) 9
Acidum Salicylicum (Salicylic Acid) 9
Aconitum Napellus (Monkswood) 10
Actaea Racemosa (Black Snake root)
(*Also known as Cimicifuga
Racemosa*) 10
Adonis Vernalis 10
Aesculus Hippocastanum (Horse
Chestnut) 10
Agaricus Muscarius (Fly Agaric) 11
Agnus Castus (Chaste Tree) 11
AIDS, Feline Syndrome Resembling
164
Aletris Farinosa (Star Grass) 11
Alimentary System, Diseases of
59–72
Allergic Contact Dermatitis 129–30
Allium Cepa (Onion) 11
Alopecia 139
Alumen (Potash Alum) 11–12
Ammonium Carbonicum
(Ammonium Carbonate) 12
Ammonium Causticum (Hydrate of
Ammonia) 12
Anaemia 124–7, 156, 157
Acute Haemorrhage-induced
124–5
Haemopoietic System
Disturbance-associated 126–7
Anaemia, Aplastic 126

Anaemia, Feline Infectious 156–7
Anaemia, Suspected 126–7
Anaphylaxis 128–9
Ankylosing Spondylitis 138
Anthracinum 12
Antimonium Arsenicosum (Arsenate
of Antimony) 13
Antimonium Crudum (Sulphide of
Antimony) 13
Antimonium Tartaricum (Tartar
Emetic) 13
Apis Mellifica (Bee Venom) 13–14
Apocynum Cannabinum (Indian
Hemp) 14
Apomorphinum 14
Appetite, Loss/Lack of 95, 132,
138, 156, 164
Appetite, Voracious 69, 70
Arching (of the Back) 95
Argentum Nitricum (Silver Nitrate)
14
Arnica Montana (Leopard's Bane)
14–15
Arsenicum Album (Arsenic Trioxide)
15
Arsenicum Iodatum (Iodide of
Arsenic) 15
Arthritis, Rheumatoid *see*
Rheumatoid (Simple) Arthritis
Ataxia, Cerebellar 153–5
Prevention (Prophylaxis) 155
Ataxia, Locomotor 89–90
Atropinum (An Alkaloid of
Belladonna) 15
Augustura Vera 12
Autonosode 5

Periosteum 135
  Damage to 142
Peritonitis, Feline Infectious *see*
  Feline Infectious Peritonitis
Petroleum (Rock Spirit) 44
Pharyngitis 61-2
Phosphoricum Acidum (Phosphoric
  Acid) 44
Phosphorus 136
Phosphorus (The Element) 44
Phytolacca Decandra (Poke Root)
  45
Platina (The Metal Platinum) 45
Pleura, Diseases of 82-6
Pleural Membranes, Inflammation of
  (Pleurisy) 85
Pleurisy 85
Pleurisy, Septic (Pyothorax) 86
Plumbum Metallicum (The Metal
  Lead) 45
Pneumonia 84-5
Pneumonitis, Feline (Chlamydial
  Infection) 150-1
Pneumonitis, Viral 84
Podophyllum (May Apple) 45
Post Partum Complications 107-10
Proctitis 67
Prostate Gland, Enlarged 110
Proteus-Bach 6-7
Psorinum (Scabies Vesicle) 46, 57
Ptelea (Water Ash) 46
Pulmonary Oedema 82-3
Pulsatilla (Anemone) 46
Pupils, Dilated 92,121
Pyelonephritis 98
Pyometra 109-10
Pyothorax 86
Pyrogenium (Artificial Sepsin) 46
Pyrogenium (Pyrogen) 57

Queen 106
  Older 109

Radial Paralysis 90-1
Ranula 60
Ranunculus Bulbosus (Buttercup) 46
Rash, Pimply 139
Rectum, Inflammation of (Proctitis)
  67
Remedy, Homoeopathic 2
  Care of 4
  Administration 3-4
  Potency Selection 3
  Preparation 2-3
Reproduction 106-11
Reproductive Systems 106-11
Rescue Remedy 47; *see also* Bach
  Flower Remedies
Respiration *see* Breathing
  (Respiration)
Respiratory System, Diseases of
  73-81
Respiratory Viruses 147-64
  Main 147-50
Reticulo-Endothelial System 145
  Attacks on 158
Retina 121-2
  Damage to 122
Retinal Detachment 121-2
Retinal Haemorrhage 121
Rheumatoid (Simple) Arthritis 138;
  see also Osteoarthritis
Rhinitis 73-4, 150
Rhino/Conjunctivitis 164
Rhododendron (Snow Rose) 47
Rhus Toxicodendron (Poison Oak)
  47
Rickets 136 – 7
Rickettsia 156
Ringworm 164
Rodent Ulcer 141
Rumex Crispus (Yellow Dock) 47
Ruta Graveolens (Rue) 47-8

Sabina (Savine) 48

Also available from Rider:

DOGS: HOMOEOPATHIC REMEDIES

George Macleod

Many dog owners today are looking for alternative ways to treat their pets when they fall ill. This book is for them. Written by a qualified veterinarian and world authority on the homoeopathic treatment of animals, this comprehensive guide introduces the key principles of homoeopathy and explains the nature of homoeopathic remedies. It includes advice on how remedies can be prepared and administered, as well as helpful information on healing the various canine bodily systems. There is practical guidance on canine viruses and bacterial diseases, including the diseases of puppyhood, making this book a must for any dog owner.

THE TREATMENT OF HORSES BY HOMOEOPATHY

George Macleod

Today, many people interested in the welfare of horses turn to treatments such as homoeopathy when their animals fall ill. This book explains how homoeopathy offers a speedy and effective means to combat equine illness, often dealing with so-called 'incurable' ailments by the use of medicines that are absolutely safe, easy to administer and which have no side effects. Written by a qualified veterinarian and world authority on the homoeopathic treatment of animals, this comprehensive guide is the culmination of many years' experience in successfully treating horses. It introduces the key principles of homoeopathy and explains the nature of homoeopathic remedies. It includes advice on how remedies can be prepared and administered, as well as helpful information on healing a wide range of equine diseases and disorders.

THE HOMOEOPATHIC TREATMENT OF SMALL ANIMALS

Principles and Practice

Christopher Day

If you would like to know more about alternative methods to treat and heal small animals, this book will set you on the right path. In this comprehensive guide, you will discover how small pets – including dogs, cats, guinea pigs, rabbits, rodents, reptiles, fish and birds – can benefit from homoeopathic remedies. There is essential information about the principles and practice of homoeopathy, as well as grounded guidance for owners, breeders and veterinary surgeons.

Helpful advice is given on getting started with the remedies, on homoeopathic first aid and on treating specific diseases. Many fascinating case studies show how homoeopathy can make an important contribution to the wellbeing of small animals.

Buy Rider Books

Order further Rider titles from your local bookshop, or have them delivered direct to your door by Bookpost